MW00604421

THE REMARKABLE TRUTH ABOUT CHIROPRACTIC

A UNIQUE JOURNEY INTO THE RESEARCH

Jeff S. Williams, DC, FIANM
AUTHOR & HOST OF THE CHIROPRACTIC FORWARD PODCAST

Cover Design: hubspot_pro
Interior Design: Nonon Tech & Design

ISBN: 978-0-578-93245-3

TABLE OF CONTENTS

INTRODUCTION

This book has been an ongoing journey. There have been times I thought it would never be completed, and there were times I thought I could finish it in a few weeks. It wound up being years before it was completed. It has absolutely been a rollercoaster.

This book had its origins back in 2008. I was building my own website and learning how to effectively market my practice. I would find interesting bits of information around the internet through sites like Yahoo Health or other similar sites. I would write a blog each week about topics such as the difference between white bread and wheat bread, or something like natural ways to reduce blood pressure. Topics such as these can be interesting; however, it wasn't what truly interested me. I'm not certain I even knew what I was interested in back then. The blogs were discussion-provoking and useful but not very focused, and other than educating the public on random topics, did not really serve much purpose in regard to practice growth.

One day I decided to find research to back up a point I was trying to make. I'm not even sure anymore what the point was, but it ultimately led me to where I am today. It was the first stone on the path I am still traveling.

By searching for a specific research topic, I started to see other related research papers. There were several papers from what I could tell and I remember being surprised. Unfortunately, I didn't know how much research was out there backing up literally everything that I do in my practice from day to day.

I thought that it might be interesting to start blogging about some of this research to let my patients know that they don't just have to take my word for it. Not only would I be learning as I waded through it, but my patients would be learning all about the research as well. It was a win-win!

Aha! That was it! I would start writing each week about research papers that support the chiropractic profession in one manner or the other. There was just one problem. I honestly thought that this task would only take me about half a year before I exhausted all the research, if it even took that long. What would I do in six months after I had exhausted all the research backing our profession?

Fortunately, "you don't know what you don't know." At this point, I must admit my former ignorance. Much to my pleasure, there turned out to be a fountain of research and information backing the chiropractic profession.

I have come to realize that the research has no end. Twelve years after I started down this road, the researchers are still keeping me in business. Not only that, it sometimes feels like I cannot keep up with the amount of information they are producing literally monthly.

I have been blogging every single week on research papers for the last several years. I still have a wealth of information in my computer I have been unable to get to. Some I will likely never get to, if I'm being truthful. This book is just a beginning. As time goes on, I suspect each section will continue to fill with fresh information in newer editions to come.

Other than an excellent research-based book by Christina L. Acompora, DC called **Marketing Chiropractic To Medical Practices**, I have yet to see a current publication with the ability to educate my colleagues, practitioners in the medical field, as well as current and potential patients. Creating one became my goal.

Clearly stated, I want to educate my colleagues. I want them to be better and more educated than I was in the first 5-10 years of my professional journey. I want them to know that they are standing on a mountain of research that says, "You are right. You've been right from the beginning. You're doing the right thing for your patients, and here's how you can prove it."

I want a book that my colleagues can use as a quick reference when approaching and communicating with medical doctors or other healthcare practitioners. Instead of giving them anecdotal evidence from their experiences, I want my fellow chiropractors to have solid, researched facts that can be clearly presented. Facts that are hard to refute even by the most old-school, hardcore chiropractic detractors.

Finally, I want current patients, as well as potential future patients to have something they can read to educate themselves. Educating themselves will allow them to make better, well-informed, evidence-based, and educated decisions for themselves and their families.

It is in that spirit that I have organized these blogs into categories. I grouped the categories in a way that I hope makes for fun and interesting reading and learning. In addition, my goal is to make the references quick and easy to find through their arrangement and categorization

As you read through this book, it may become painfully apparent that I am not an author by trade. This is for two reasons:
1. I am not an author.
2. I have made a very direct effort to write these blogs in a way that **ANYONE** can read through them, learn from them, and process the information. Not only can anyone read it, but also **UNDERSTAND** it. One cannot accomplish this feat (in my opinion) by using big words and difficult techno-babble phrases that only a person in the healthcare or the research field can comprehend.

The information within is research- and evidence-based. If I want to maintain open dialogue with those in the medical profession and foster an atmosphere of cooperation, the use or promotion of chiropractic jargon or terminology is better left out.

While the medical field is not generally aware of common chiropractic terminology, they are much more accepting and open to us when we speak in terms of research. These are terms they understand clearly. For instance, if you try to speak to an orthopedic surgeon about the concepts of chiropractic philosophy for 30 minutes, no matter your conviction to the concept, you are likely going to be talking to a blank stare. This defeats the overall purpose.

However, if you show the same individual peer-reviewed, randomized controlled trials having to do with the successful treatment of low back pain through spinal mobilization or manipulation, then you are going to have a much more accepting audience. You will dramatically lessen your workload when communicating in the language they speak every day.

It has been my experience that promoting the treatment of **non**-neuromusculoskeletal conditions is **not** helpful in achieving the goal of wider chiropractic utilization. It is my opinion that we must show that we belong as part of mainstream healthcare. We must do this through use of the research that has already been done. It's just sitting there waiting for us to use it more effectively. I don't mean just any research though. I mean randomized controlled trials, systematic reviews, meta-analyses; high-quality research - NOT biased, pilot or case studies, and certainly not any of those performed by stakeholders with something to gain from a favorable outcome.

Many of my colleagues will disagree with my opinion and I fully expect the discussion. However, it is just that: my opinion. It is how I run my practice. It is how I communicate with others. It is how I mentor and teach others.

Although anecdotal evidence has value, it is still only anecdotal and proves little. Recognizing this, I choose to stand on proof, evidence, and research instead. Doing so is certainly an effective way to approach our patients and laypeople in general. Once you transfer the language into the correct vernacular, then you are communicating effectively.

WHAT THIS BOOK IS NOT.

Readers will come across profession comparisons in this book. This book is not an attempt to bash the medical profession as a whole. It is not to run down the education of other professions in the interest of promoting chiropractic. It is not to denigrate any profession. However, in advocating for the chiropractic profession, comparisons to competitors and competing techniques is next to impossible.

The overall goal is simply to say:
- We evidence-based, patient-centered chiropractors are good at what we do,
- We are highly educated healthcare practitioners,
- We use conservative and cost-effective techniques,
- We deserve the respect that we have earned and continue to earn every single day,
- We have very well-thought and well-researched solutions to the most common neuromusculoskeletal conditions,
- We deserve a seat at the table of conventional healthcare, and
- We have research backing all of it up!

ACKNOWLEDGEMENTS

I have a lot of people to thank for sending me on this journey. Some family, some inspirations, some friendly, and some foe.

I want to start with God. I've been blessed in more ways than I can even begin to describe and I am shown these blessings all the time. I am constantly grateful.

My family. My beautiful wife, Meg. She is literally one of the smartest people I've ever met in my life (if not THE smartest). She has been my rock, my advisor, my confidante, my person to worry with, my person to celebrate with, my person to turn to for every emotion good or bad, and my best friend. My person.

My kids. Jake and Joss have put up with their Dad not getting home until after dark. They've put up with their Mom and Dad being at work till late at night doing payroll, special events, etc. while they wonder what we're having for dinner. I love you both infinitely and am proud of you both.

My Mom, Sheryl, was the one that told me I could be anything I wanted to be and was there to support me in everything I ever attempted with an encouraging word and a kind and gentle smile. My Mom is the one that set up my first chiropractic visit in Perryton, TX when I was a freshman in high school and had injured myself skiing.

My brother, my Dad, my Step-Dads, my grandparents, and anyone else who helped light a fire of some sort and/or foster a talent they saw within me.

Professionally I want to thank my colleagues I look to daily for information, advice, and inspiration.

I want to thank Dr. Chris Howson, inventor of the Drop Release tool (www.droprelease.com) located in Grand Forks, ND and Dr. Steven Roffers located of Chiropractic Research Alliance located in Palm Springs, CA for helping me with the editing process.

Thank you to the business associates I have dealt with through the years that have made me want to learn and achieve more. Whether it was through your kindness or through your obstacles, I grew stronger and persevered because of you. Thanks to all that played a part.

RESEARCH STANDARDS & BEST PRACTICES

As alluded to previously, in the world of research, there are different levels of information and different levels of the value that information truly holds. As I stated in the beginning of this book, these papers were originally presented in a blog format so they do not look all that "scientific" when presented here in this format. However, some basic knowledge of research papers and protocol is necessary if one decides to use a research citation to track down the full paper.

In addition, there will be many times in which the citation states, "This was a randomized controlled trial," or, "This paper was a meta-analysis," or something similar. Basic knowledge of research terminology will help you to understand more thoroughly what you are reading.

In the image below, you will see how the studies become more and more rigorous the further up the pyramid you ascend. The papers offer less chance for bias and are more reliable in general.

This general guideline will help you to better discern the quality of paper you are reviewing.

With help from Duke University[1], I also feel it is beneficial to provide quick descriptions of the different types of studies for a comprehensive understanding:

1. **Case Series/Case Reports** – these are a grouping of different reports on treatments of various people. It could also be a report on a specific individual. Due to the lack of a control group, they tend to have low reliability.

2. **Case Control Studies** - researchers take a condition, they take patients that already have the condition, and then they compare them to individuals who do not have the condition. The authors will try to figure out what the patients with the condition may, or may not, have been exposed to. In simpler terms: why these people are suffering from it while these others are not. This type of study is still not as reliable as randomized controlled trials.
3. **Cohort Studies** – this type of study accepts patients that are undergoing a certain treatment for a condition. The authors will continue following the subjects over a specified amount of time eventually comparing their results with those of a group of subjects that were not undergoing the treatment.
4. **Randomized Controlled Clinical Trials** – these studies are well-planned. They typically implement means to reduce any chance of author bias and typically include comparison between the treatment group and a control group. Randomized controlled trials are generally considered to be fairly reliable.
5. **Systematic Reviews** – these studies typically focus on a topic and aim to answer a specific question pertaining to the topic. They normally include an exhaustive literature search taken from databases commonly used by research authors such as MEDLINE and EMBASE. After the authors determine which papers will be accepted into the systematic review, they are reviewed, the quality is determined, and they are then summarized into a reasonable conclusion.
6. **Meta-Analysis** – a complete examination of a particular topic using valid studies accepted under standardized and commonly-used protocols to summarize them into one paper.

Obviously, this is a top-down, macro view of research papers and the various types of research. In reality, the research world is much more intricate and complicated, but this is a good start with simple, basic concepts that will likely clear up questions that may arise as one progresses through this book.

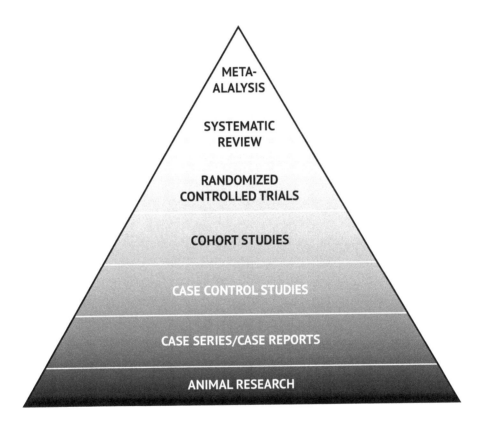

WILK VS. AMERICAN MEDICAL ASSOCIATION (AMA)

When making the case for chiropractic's legitimacy, I think it is reasonable to start with the Wilk vs. AMA case. The facts of this case are truly stunning when you think about them and dive down into the information. When viewed from a current day perspective, it is hard to imagine.

The American Medical Association made it their mission to completely obliterate the chiropractic profession from the United States of America and, hopefully, the world. I truly doubt there would be a need for a book like this without a sustained, consistent, century-long attack on chiropractic by the AMA.

As mentioned in the introduction, I am not putting down the medical profession when speaking about this case. The truth is, most medical doctors are members of the AMA but most medical doctors have no idea, nor do they have the time to care, what the AMA does on their behalf. For the good OR for the bad. They are simply, for the most part, unaware.

Four chiropractors and Chester Wilk sued the AMA in 1976. The lawsuit alleged that the AMA and others were guilty of antitrust. Specifically, the claim was that the AMA was responsible for years and years of coordinated and illegal, conspiratorial attacks on the chiropractic profession in an attempt to contain and ultimately eliminate the profession.

In 1987, after 11 years of legal wrangling, a judge in a federal appellate court ruled the AMA did in fact engage in a "lengthy, systematic, successful and unlawful boycott" concerning chiropractors and the chiropractic profession. The proceedings proved the AMA coordinated attacks in the following ways:

- They tried to undermine chiropractic schools.
- Medical doctors were not allowed to teach at chiropractic colleges or to even speak where chiropractors were gathered.
- They actively attempted to contain chiropractic schools.
- They discouraged colleges, universities, and faculty from cooperating with chiropractic schools.
- They tried to knowingly keep evidence of the effectiveness of chiropractic care from public knowledge.
- They said it was unethical for medical doctors to associate with chiropractors.
- They labeled chiropractic as an unscientific cult.
- The AMA created a committee on quackery specifically to undermine chiropractic.
- They disallowed medical doctors from referring to chiropractors.
- They disallowed medical doctors from **accepting referrals** from chiropractors.
- They likened chiropractors to "killers and rabid dogs."
- They enticed other healthcare and medical organizations and associations to sign on to their chiropractic boycott.
- They were able to force non-AMA members to abide by their new regulations by getting the hospital associations to require following them. They did this through the Joint Commission on Accreditation of Hospitals as well as through the American College of Physicians. The medical doctors were to follow the rules and get in line or lose hospital privileges regardless of whether they were members of the AMA or not.
- They organized, printed, and distributed anti-chiropractic literature.
- They helped other organizations print and distribute literature critical of chiropractic.

- They encouraged complaints against doctors of chiropractic based on lack of ethics.
- They actively opposed any chiropractic inroads into insurance.
- They actively opposed chiropractic inroads in Workmen's Compensation.
- They actively opposed chiropractic inroads into labor unions.
- They actively opposed chiropractic inroads into hospitals.

They did all of this damage through cooperation with other organizations as well as through the state medical associations down the chain. The state medical associations then dispersed the information to the individual medical doctors practicing in the field. Today, in the times we live in, this doesn't even sound like a real possibility. Yet, it is a fact and it is in court record.

As I stated, the AMA was found guilty in 1987. Specifically, they were found guilty of violating section 1, but not section 2, of the Sherman Anti-Trust act, and had, in fact, played a part in the illegal restraint of trade against the chiropractic profession. Not only that, but the judge also added in her comments that the AMA "had entered into a long history of illegal behavior." But that wasn't the end of the story.

Following the decision in 1987, after both sides appealed the decision, the original ruling was upheld by the US Court of Appeals in February 1990. Of course, the AMA petitioned the US Supreme Court three more times, but each petition was denied a hearing.

This is a fairly quick summary. There are certainly much more in-depth and detailed descriptions concerning this case. However, what I have stated here is enough to make the layperson understand the need, even today, for a book such as this.

Although the two professions enjoy much more cooperation, camaraderie, and integration in the present day, the lingering effects of this decades-long campaign of hate are still painfully obvious. They are obvious in online chat rooms and discussions. They are still obvious when every now and then, our patients come back to us after a visit to an unfriendly family doctor. The lingering effects are most certainly still present to this day.

For a more current example of the lingering effects, during an election cycle in 2014, a Texas chiropractor ran for a local office in Austin, TX. The Texas Medical Association PAC continued waging this campaign of hate when they mailed postcards to the households in the chiropractor's district. One side of the postcard asked the commonalities shared by Dr. Hyde, Dr. Pepper, and a Dr. Of Chiropractic. The snarky response to the questions was that none of them held a medical degree.

Even worse, the other side was filled with the image of a huge duck. The words read, "Quack, quack, quack."

Let me be clear: this type of attack still goes on in certain circles of the medical profession. Can you imagine where chiropractic would be today if not for this shameful hate campaign against chiropractic? I wonder how many people have suffered from pain that a chiropractor could have easily treated?

GENERAL DISCUSSION

While it is true that chiropractic is presently more respected and better poised to integrate into mainstream healthcare than at any time in the past, there are still many battles left to fight. I will take this portion of the book to simply share history, experience, thoughts, and opinions.

As I type, I am the Department Chair for the Texas Chiropractic Association's (TCA) Scientific Affairs Committee. In that capacity, and in some ten years serving on the TCA Board - as its Public Relations Chairman, and as its Chiropractic Development Initiative Chairman - I have seen the defeat of one seven-year long legal attack on our right to diagnose from the Texas Medical Association (TMA) only to be followed up by a subsequent lawsuit by the TMA on our right to perform vestibulo-ocular nystagmus testing (VONT) with special training. They tried to figure out a way to tie that issue back into the Diagnosis complaint therefore, we ended up with a "Diagnosis: Part Two" trial.

The second case was just recently won by Texas chiropractors when the Texas Supreme Court ruled in favor of Texas Chiropractors on all accounts. The TCA and the Texas Board of Chiropractic Examiners (TBCE) ultimately prevailed after yet another, financially draining, seven-year battle.

Also, in more recent sessions of the Texas Legislature, the TMA has continued attacking the chiropractic profession. If they cannot win through the courts, they seem to be determined to win through legislation and they have physicians in seats of Congress to help them along the way.

They have attacked chiropractors' right to perform simple school exams. This is a right chiropractors have enjoyed for generations with no complaints and no children being harmed as a result of a chiropractor having performed the exam.

In addition, the TMA has spearheaded efforts to prevent chiropractors from serving on the Medical Advisory Committee for the Concussion Oversight Team in Texas. To put that in perspective, athletic trainers are allowed on the Committee.

As part of the continued assault on chiropractic, the TMA continues to oppose chiropractors' right to perform simple exams on bus drivers. Chiropractors have been performing exams on truck drivers and heavy equipment operators for years. Chiropractors even go through additional training and nationally accepted certification specifically for this sort of examination.

In addition, the TMA recently opposed chiropractors having the ability to issue simple handicapped placards so that their injured patients, those that have Multiple Sclerosis, advanced arthritis or degeneration, or difficulty with gait, can get a better parking spot.

I believe, after reviewing the charts in the education comparison section, it is clear that chiropractors can adequately and confidently make a proper evaluation as to a patient's handicap status.

Let us talk about musculoskeletal treatment in general. Medical doctors and the medical field as a whole have never seriously come up with a good answer for musculoskeletal treatment. Think about it; what happens when one goes to a medical provider for muscle strains, sprains, joint pain, neck pain, or low back pain? It has been my experience that, typically, a patient will be given one, or a combination of, the following:
1. Muscle relaxants
2. Pain pills
3. Anti-inflammatories

If it is deemed serious enough or one of the above does not take care of the issue, the patient may be kicked down the line to a physical therapist for treatment. As with any profession, there are good and bad members. PT is a wonderful answer for post-operative rehab, certain injuries, and prevention of scar tissue buildup. However, PT is not the answer in all cases, and it has been shown through research that PT is not as effective as chiropractic manipulation/mobilization in many cases. In fact, in more recent research, chiropractic has bested PT and care with a primary care physician in the categories for patient satisfaction, outcomes, and being the more cost-effective treatment.

As you read this book, it will become more and more obvious that chiropractic is getting intentionally kicked to the wayside and excluded from the chain of care regardless of continued research showing the amazing benefits and effectiveness of what we do.

One of the more recent attacks included attacks against a chiropractor's right to diagnose their patients. Meaning, we will no longer be "portal of entry" practitioners. We would only be able to treat what the medical doctors send us to treat. I think it is clear how that would turn out for the chiropractor working out in the field.

The Affordable Care Act (ACA) has had some negatives to it. However, there was a positive aspect to the ACA. Or so we thought. The part of the ACA that chiropractors looked forward to was Section 2706.

Section 2706 of the ACA is also called the "Nondiscrimination Health Care" section and was written by Senator Tom Harkin (D-Iowa). The wording basically says that chiropractors (and others qualified) are to be paid equally for the services they perform as those more "conventional" disciplines such as medical doctors, osteopaths, physical therapists, are paid.

It sounds silly to say but it is common that a medical physician, a nurse practitioner, physician assistant, or physical therapist will get reimbursed at a higher rate than a chiropractor for the exact same physical exam or evaluation. Chiropractors are equally trained, if not more trained, in physical exam, evaluation, and diagnosis of Neuromusculoskeletal conditions but are paid less for the same work.

Section 2706 was meant to level the playing field a bit. However, that has not been the case. In fact, as far as my colleagues and I can tell, nothing has changed at all. In fact, a good argument could be made that the ACA has made things worse on chiropractors. Since its inception, premiums have doubled, co-pays have doubled, deductibles have doubled, and insurance companies have reduced the levels they reimburse doctors.

It has been stated that the AMA's #2 goal is the elimination of Section 2706. Why would that be? Sen. Harkin has retired, there is no enforcement of this section at the national level, and there is zero enforcement at the state level. We are a nation of laws, but it appears this law has no teeth from what I have seen thus far.

In the end, it is my humble opinion that the real loser in this turf war is the patient. I believe that a concerted, cooperative, and integrated approach to care is the optimum treatment available. Chiropractic is not the answer to all problems. At the same time, neither are pills and injections. There should be an ongoing discussion in regard to medicine integrating with complementary and alternative means of treatment.

Can chiropractic help a person control migraines? There is research suggesting that it can. Can a combination of chiropractic, therapeutic massage, and acupuncture keep the migraines at bay even more effectively? Are those not questions to be asking rather than simply performing injections into the suboccipital region followed by a lifetime of pills to try to control the migraines? I have seen several patients throughout the years that this was the answer they were given before discovering chiropractic on their own.

To continue with my example of migraines and headaches, I think the preferred treatment for chronic and debilitating migraines should be completion of a Headache Disability Questionnaire (HDQ) Assessment, a short trial of chiropractic treatment with a 2-4 week re-exam to assess effectiveness through another HDQ. If effectiveness is minor, implement therapeutic massage and acupuncture, complete a follow-up HDQ in another 4 weeks. If there is still only mild improvement, implement traditional medical means.

Obviously, I am glossing over some steps and details. In general, we see approximately 70%-80% of tension-type headaches and (to a lesser extent) migraines and headaches improve greatly from chiropractic mobilization and soft tissue work alone. I realize that is not very convenient for those selling headache and migraine medications, but it is extremely advantageous and cost-effective for patients.

Chiropractic is not a modality. Present-day chiropractic is not just 'popping bones' and sending them home. Present-day chiropractic is a profession. A profession with an umbrella that includes the following for example:
- Spinal manipulative therapy
- Exercise/Rehabilitation
- Acupuncture
- Massage/Soft Tissue Manipulation
- Physiotherapy modalities
- Proprioceptive/Balance training
- Sports preparation/recovery
- Low-level laser
- Non-surgical decompression
- Biomechanics training

It should definitely be a part of the discussion if our highest priority is the care of the patient. If ethics and the Hippocratic Oath hold true, chiropractic will be in this discussion at a higher level in the future.

Speaking of the **Hippocratic Oath**, I have picked out the parts of the modern version that easily apply to the implementation of chiropractic treatment for conventional therapy:

- I will apply, for the benefit of the sick, **all measures required**, avoiding those twin traps of over treatment and therapeutic nihilism.
- I will remember that there is art to medicine as well as science, and that warmth, sympathy, and understanding **may outweigh the surgeon's knife or the chemist's drug.**
- I will not be ashamed to say, "I know not," **nor will I fail to call in my colleagues when the skills of another are needed for a patient's recovery.**
- I will prevent disease whenever I can, for **prevention is preferable to cure.**

Can you see where the medical field, insurance companies, and stakeholders can improve?

Hopefully, this book can aid in beginning an honest dialogue and be an impetus toward real opportunities to work together in cooperation and to integrate evidence-based, patient-centered chiropractic treatment into the conventional model of healthcare.

Now, onto the research!

EDUCATION COMPARISONS

I want to make something very clear: my goal is not to denigrate other professions. My goal is to prove the validity of chiropractic.

The listed hours represent the standard curriculum at institutions. The graphs do not take into account continued personal achievement or continuing education beyond their curriculum completion[2].

Data can be independently verified and was collected from 2016 academic calendars among the top ranked programs in North America.

Professions in the graphs are listed as follows:
- DC – Doctor of Chiropractic – (4614 hrs.) University of Western States
- MD – Medical Doctor – (4800 hrs.) Yale School of Medicine
- DO – Doctor of Osteopathy – (4600 hrs.) Touro College of Osteopathic Medicine
- DPT – Doctor of Physical Therapy – (2667 hrs.) University of Southern California

Specific programs at different institutions will vary; charts are provided for basic comparison and education priorities of each profession, and not imply any one profession is 'better' than another. Please recognize that while education plays a role in practice style, the charts below do not take into consideration post graduate education, practice preference, or clinical specialization.

In online discussions, I have seen people denigrating the education of chiropractors. They agree that chiropractors get a lot of hours, but they say they are not quality classes. I firmly disagree.

Chiropractic schools are accredited through the Council on Chiropractic Education (CCE) which is recognized by the Council for Higher Education Accreditation (CHEA) and is a member of the Association specialized and Professional Accreditors (ASPA).

In addition, many of the professors in chiropractic colleges are medical doctors, chiropractic doctors, as well as PhDs. A chiropractic student must undergo the same basic science courses as any medical student must undergo. These courses include Cell Biology, Systemic Anatomy, Gross Anatomy (I & II), Biochemistry (I & II), Microbiology/Immunology, Public Health, General Pathology, Systems Pathology, Radiology (I, II, & III), Clinical Orthopedics, Lab Diagnosis, Clinical Neurology, Physiology (I, II, and III), Emergency Care, Differential Diagnosis, Internship, and much more.

When you experience people diminishing Chiropractic Education, recognize it for what it is: ignorance of the topic.

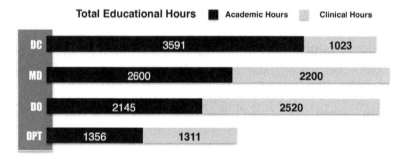

Total Educational Hours ■ Academic Hours ▨ Clinical Hours

	Academic Hours	Clinical Hours
DC	3591	1023
MD	2600	2200
DO	2145	2520
DPT	1356	1311

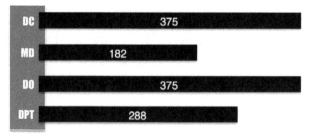

Anatomy Educational Hours

	Hours
DC	375
MD	182
DO	375
DPT	288

Jeff S. Williams, DC, FIANM

Diagnostic Imaging Educational Hours

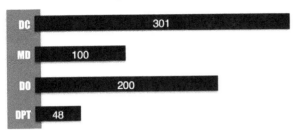

Physiology Educational Hours

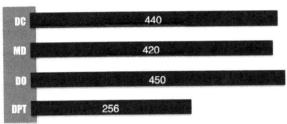

Orthopaedics Educational Hours

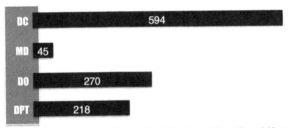

Soft Tissue Mobilization Educational Hours

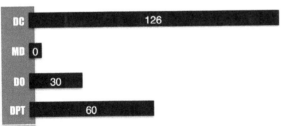

Rehab & Exercise Educational Hours

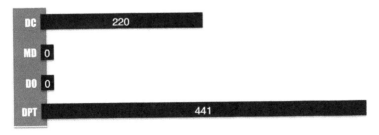

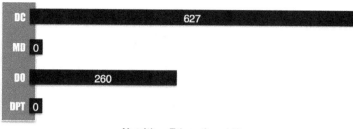

Nutrition Educational Hours

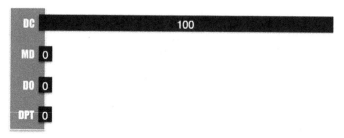

Here are more graphics demonstrating the thoroughness of chiropractic education. These are via Texas Chiropractic Association. Again, totals do not take into account post-graduate work, residencies, etc.

Chiropractic Student Hours	Class Description	Medical Student Hours
520	Anatomy	508
420	Physiology	326
271	Pathology	335
300	Chemistry	325
114	Bacteriology	130
370	Diagnosis	374
320	Neurology	112
217	X-Ray	148
65	Pyschiatry	144
65	Obstetrics & Gynecology	198
225	Orthopedics	156
2,887	**Total Hours**	**2,756**
1,598	Speciality Courses	1,492
4,485	**Entire Total Hours**	**4,248**

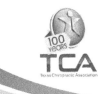

Healthcare Education Comparison

	TEXAS★STATE UNIVERSITY	TEXAS	UTPA	TEXAS TECH UNIVERSITY HEALTH SCIENCES CENTER	TEXAS TECH UNIVERSITY HEALTH SCIENCES CENTER	TEX★S Chiropractic College
	Athletic Trainer	Family Nurse Practitioner	Physician's Assistant	Doctor of Physical Therapy	Medical Doctor	Doctor of Chiropractic
Admissions	High School Diploma Minimum GPA 2.75	Bachelor's Degree in Nursing Minimum GPA 3.0	Pre-requisites: 33 undergraduate hours GPA of ≥3.0	Bachelor's Degree in Minimum GPA 3.0	Bachelor's Degree 90 semester hours, GPA 3.6 or greater, MCAT of 30	Bachelor's Degree 90 semester hours, GPA 3.0 or greater, MCAT N/A
Total Collegiate Years	4 Years	5 Years	5 Years	7 Years	8 Years	8 Years
Credit Hours Post Bachelor's Degree	0 Credit Hours	41 Credit Hours	100 Credit Hours	100 Credit Hours	160 Credit Hours	220 Credit Hours
Residency and Clinical Rotations	480 Clock Hours (about 12 weeks)	180 Clock Hours (about 4 ½ weeks)	32 Weeks	32 Weeks	3-8 Years Depending on Specialty	1 Year Clinical Rounds Residency
References	www.txstate.edu	nursing.uth.edu	www.utpa.edu	www.ttuhsc.edu	www.ttuhsc.edu/som	www.txchiro.edu

SOMETHING YOU PROBABLY HAVEN'T BEEN TOLD ABOUT CHIROPRACTIC EDUCATION

This entry helps to spotlight the advanced capabilities of chiropractic students. Also, there are some quick to dismiss the idea of a chiropractor serving in the role of a primary care provider. The idea may not be as far-fetched as they might have you believe.

Let us consider some things. We hear repeatedly that there is a shortage of physicians. We are witnessing physician assistants and nurse practitioners gaining more and more scope and ability as the years pass in an effort to fill the void.

In addition, with more stress, electronic health record demands, and documentation demands, many in the medical field are choosing to retire early.

One can also take into consideration the rise in popularity of alternative healthcare options. Considering all factors, it is my argument that the chiropractic profession has the ability to step up its game and help fill the gaps that will eventually be left.

This research paper suggests that there would be very little work left to do in regard to getting chiropractic students up to speed and ready for them to fulfill the primary care role.

Why they did it

The authors' stated research goal was to take a closer look at chiropractic education and chiropractic students' knowledge of primary care tasks in comparison to their counterparts in the medical schools.

How They Did It

- Three samples of chiropractic student were used versus one sample of medical students.
- They were given tests regarding the knowledge of primary care tasks
- The tests were given to final term chiropractic students as well as medical students that were entering their residency programs

What They Found

- The chiropractic students scored below the medical students on the exam in every area except for the musculoskeletal conditions.
- The chiropractors scored higher than the medical students on the musculoskeletal portion.

Wrap It Up

In this paper, while medical students did score better in all aspects other than the musculoskeletal portion, it is to be noted that the chiropractic students performed almost as well.

Basically, if medical school is what we measure primary care education by, then the fact that chiropractic students scored almost as well as the medical students is worth spotlighting, recognizing, realizing, and discussing[3].

WHAT YOU SHOULD KNOW ABOUT CHIROPRACTIC, MEDICAL DOCTORS, AND RADIOLOGY

I know the educational regimen and requirements that my colleagues and I went through. Our education, much like the education of medical doctors or osteopaths, is a full-time job. When taking 33 hours in just one semester, there is truly little time for anything else, including family.

As mentioned previously, it needs to be pointed out that any time I highlight educational points for chiropractors and educational requirements of other professions, it is never to denigrate other professions. I truly believe that the patient wins when there is a combined effort in the treatment protocol. I highly respect and value all healthcare professions and practitioners. Current research is teaching us that the best treatment is a multimodal approach utilize several tools in the toolbox rather than just one hammer.

The goal is to contrast and compare education levels so that the reader and healthcare consumer can be better educated and make a more informed decision.

Why They Did It

The authors' stated objectives in this study were to compare medical students and chiropractic students by testing their knowledge when evaluating x-ray images of the low back spine and of the pelvis. Although low back pain, and resulting radiology studies, continues to be a large part of healthcare complaints and emergency room visits, there has never been a comparison of the practitioners that are likely to be the ones reading these x-rays.

How They Did It
- This paper was a controlled comparison of x-ray interpretation based on experience and training.
- 496 volunteers
- The volunteers were from nine target groups
- Participants completed a test of x-ray interpretation
- The exam had 19 cases all with important x-ray findings
- The nine groups consisted of 22 medical students, 183 chiropractic students, 27 medical radiology residents, 13 chiropractic radiology residents, 66 medical clinicians, 46 chiropractic clinician's, 48 general medical radiologists, 55 chiropractic radiologists, and 36 skeletal radiologists and fellows

What They Found
- There were significant differences found among the professional groups.
- Skeletal radiologists had significantly better testing than all other medical groups
- The test results were better for general medical radiologists and medical radiology residents than for those of medical clinicians
- The results for the medical students were significantly poorer than all of the other medical groups.
- There was no difference in the performance of chiropractic clinicians and chiropractic students
- **The test results for the chiropractic radiologists, the chiropractic radiology residents, and the chiropractic students were significantly higher than that of the corresponding medical categories.**
- Also, there was no significant difference in the testing results between **chiropractic radiologists and skeletal radiologists.**

Wrap It Up

All that needs to be repeated considering these results is the fact that the test results for chiropractic radiologists, chiropractic radiology residents, and chiropractic students were significantly higher than that of the corresponding medical categories. Also, there was no difference between the chiropractic radiologists and skeletal radiologists. Considering the skeletal radiologists were the best of all other medical groups, Chiropractic radiologists, by default, were also better than all other medical groups.

What that means in my interpretation is that you would rather have a chiropractor reading your x-ray images when given the option.[4]

HOW MUCH DOES THE RUN-OF-THE-MILL MEDICAL STUDENT KNOW ABOUT TREATING MUSCULOSKELETAL ISSUES?

Before I get into this paper, I want to share a story of my own.

I went to the emergency room several years ago. I had diagnosed myself with three different issues. I had a pretty good idea of what was going on, but I decided to go just as a precaution.

I'm getting to that age where the ticker can get sketchy on some guys, so I wanted to play it safe and make sure it wasn't getting funny on ME! Anyway, I told the ER doctor that I felt like I had a bulged/herniated disc. He pushed down on my head to test, but that was about all that he did. My disc testing and classification system in my clinic is leaps and bounds more advanced than the average ER physician! I have at least five different orthopedic tests for a disc in the cervical spine.

Eventually, he was honest enough to say, "You'd probably know better than me if it's a disc." I thought that was great to get a little credit from a physician. He was good and very thorough on what he knew and what he was comfortable with. I am not trying to disrespect him here. I think he was very competent on what he has been taught.

But, according to research, he is 100% correct.

Why They Did It
A basic understanding of the musculoskeletal system is essential when practicing medicine. It made sense to the authors to survey a portion of healthcare practitioners try to assess the level of understanding of the musculoskeletal system.

How Did They Do It?
- An exam was issued to 334 volunteers
- The volunteers had to be medical students, residents, and/or staff physicians.

What Did They Find?
The average score was a 57%
- 69 of the 334 (21%) scored a 73.1 or higher
- Of the 69 people that scored a 73.1 or higher, 58% of those were orthopedic residents and staff physicians.

Wrap It Up
79% of the participants failed the basic musculoskeletal cognitive examination suggesting that training in the realm of the musculoskeletal system is woefully inadequate in medical school as well as non-orthopedic residency programs[5].

CHIROPRACTIC UTILIZATION STUDIES

CHIROPRACTIC CARE IN PRIMARY PREVENTION

Effect of chiropractic treatment on primary or early secondary prevention: a systematic review with a pedagogic approach" by Goncalves, et. al[6] and published in Chiropractic and Manual Therapies in 2018.

Why They Did It
The chiropractic vitalistic approach to the concept of 'subluxation' as a cause of disease lacks both biological plausibility and possibly proof of validity. Nonetheless, some chiropractors purport to prevent disease in general through chiropractic care. Evidence of this effect is needed to be allowed to continue this practice. The objective of this systematic review was to investigate for evidence that spinal manipulations/chiropractic care can be used in primary prevention (PP) and/or early secondary prevention in diseases other than musculoskeletal conditions.

How They Did It
- As the title gives away, it's a systematic review, which indicates more dependable information. Systematic reviews lie at the top of the research pyramid.
- They searched PubMed, Embase, Index to Chiropractic Literature, and specialized chiropractic journals from inception all the way up to October 2017

- For the search, they used terms like chiropractic, subluxation, prevention, wellness, spinal manipulation, and mortality.
- They included anything mentioning the study of the clinical preventative effect or benefit from manipulative therapy or chiropractic treatment in relation to primary prevention or the treatment of physical disease in general. Anything other than musculoskeletal disorders.
- Population studies were also eligible
- Checklists were designed in relation to the description of the reviewed articles and some basic quality criteria.

What They Found
- Of the 13.099 titles scrutinized, 13 articles were included (eight clinical studies and five population studies).
- These studies dealt with various disorders of public health importance such as diastolic blood pressure, blood test immunological markers, and mortality.
- Only two clinical studies could be used for data synthesis. None showed any effect of spinal manipulation/chiropractic treatment.

Wrap It Up
The authors concluded by saying, "We found no evidence in the literature of an effect of chiropractic treatment in the scope of PP or early secondary prevention for disease in general. Chiropractors have to assume their role as evidence-based clinicians and the leaders of the profession must accept that it is harmful to the profession to imply public health importance in relation to the prevention of such diseases through manipulative therapy/chiropractic treatment."

CHIROPRACTIC WITH MEDICAL CARE IS MORE EFFECTIVE THAN MEDICAL CARE BY ITSELF

Chiropractic treatment in conjunction with traditional medical treatment has shown to provide more relief than medical care alone according to new research.

Why They Did It
The authors wanted to know what the combination of the two methods (Medical and Chiropractic) would produce and if it made sense to support it.

How They Did It
- They took 91 military personnel with low back pain
- All received traditional medical care
- 50% of the group also received chiropractic adjustments

What They Found
1. 73% of the chiropractic group experienced moderate and above moderate relief from pain
2. 17% of the control group experienced the same level of relief as the chiropractic group
3. Chiropractic also had disability scores that were far lower than the control group

Wrap It Up
There's no doubt here. There is a clear advantage when using chiropractic treatment in addition to traditional healthcare[7].

RESEARCHED & TESTED TREATMENT FOR LONG-TERM PAIN

Why They Did It

The authors of this paper wanted to find out the efficacy of medication, acupuncture, and spinal manipulation in long-term (chronic) conditions

How They Did It
- The study was a randomized clinical trial.
- The study took place at Townsville's General Hospital from 1999-2001.
- The study ran for 9 weeks.
- 69 subjects were treated by the various protocols.
- They were assessed and followed-up on a full year after treatment was concluded.
- The Outcome Assessments used were Oswestry Back Pain Index, Neck Disability index, Short-Form-36, and Visual Analogue Scale.

What They Found
- For the spinal manipulation group, there was absolute efficacy shown in the Outcome Assessment measurements.
- For chiropractic treatment, there was a broad-based long-term benefit in 5 of the 7 outcome measures.
- There was only ONE outcome measure showing efficacy in the acupuncture and in the medication group.

Wrap It Up

"In patients with chronic spinal pain syndromes, spinal manipulation, if not contraindicated, may be the only treatment modality of the assessed regimens that provides broad and significant long-term benefit[8]."

CHIROPRACTIC WINS THE CHALLENGE FOR LOW BACK PAIN

Why They Did It

The authors wanted to compare hospital outpatient care with chiropractic for low back pain treatment.

How They Did It
- This paper was a randomized comparison.
- The study consisted of 741 men and women.
- The subjects were aged 18-64.
- The Outcome Assessments were performed via the Oswestry questionnaire.

What They Found
- At the three-year mark, there was a 29% greater improvement in the subjects treated via chiropractic over those treated by the hospital outpatient regimen.
- Chiropractic was particularly effective for pain. Patients rated chiropractic as the more helpful protocol at the three-year mark.

Wrap It Up

"At three years the results confirm the findings of an earlier report that when chiropractic or hospital therapists treat patients with low back pain as they would in day to day practice those treated by chiropractic derive more benefit and long term satisfaction than those treated by hospitals[9]."

REFLEX RESPONSES AFTER CHIROPRACTIC ADJUSTMENTS

Why They Did It

The goal of this paper was to try to find out what kind of reflex response is elicited from a spinal manipulation (chiropractic adjustment).

How They Did It

- 10 men without any symptoms were used.
- 11 spinal manipulative treatments were administered along the full length of the spine.
- 16 bipolar surface electrodes placed strategically measured the reflex responses.

What They Found

- Each chiropractic adjustment showed reflex responses in the area the adjustment targeted.
- The responses happened within 50-200 msec after the adjustment.
- The reflex responses lasted for 100-400 msec in duration.

Wrap It Up

"This is the first study in which results show a consistent reflex response associated with spinal manipulative treatments. Because reflex pathways are evoked systematically during spinal manipulative treatment, there is a distinct possibility that these responses may cause some of the clinically observed beneficial effects, such as a reduction in pain and a decrease in hypertonicity of muscles[10]."

EVER HAD A CHIROPRACTOR TELL YOU TO COME BACK?

Why They Did It

The authors were curious as to whether there was any real, measured benefit to continued "maintenance" or "wellness" visits **beyond the initial phase of care** in regard to CHRONIC low back pain.

It's a great question that needed to be asked because patients come into our offices concerned about having to come see a chiropractor a million times, etc. Is there any real benefit?

How They Did It
1. Single blinded, placebo-controlled
2. 60 patients
3. All chronic
4. They had to have suffered from the pain for at least 6 months.
5. Randomized to receive either
   - 12 adjustments of fake treatment over a 1-month period or
   - 12 treatments of actual treatments over a 1-month period with no treatment in the following nine months.
   - 12 treatments of actual treatments over a 1-month period followed by manipulation every 2 weeks for the next 9 months.

They measured pain and disability scores, generic health status, and back-specific patient satisfaction at 1, 4, 7 and 10-month intervals.

What They Found

Patients in the manipulation groups had significantly less pain and disability than did the first group when the 1-month period was up.

Only the third group (the one with follow up maintenance treatment) showed more improvement in these scores at the 10-month evaluation.

Wrap It Up

This study indicates that maintenance spinal manipulation offers the best long-term benefit[11].

COMPARISON OF COMBINED APPROACH TO ACUTE LOW BACK PAIN – 2011

This study was held in the UK in 2011 so the information is recent. The study makes mention of a "stratified" primary care management protocol. This term is used to describe the use of alternative treatment (manual therapy).

As one reads through this paper, it would be appropriate to replace the word "stratified" with alternative treatments or manual therapy.

How They Did It

The authors understood back pain remains a significant challenge for primary practitioners to treat and manage. They were also aware of the fact that co-management of back pain among primary practitioners and alternative therapies had not yet been tested.

How They Did It.

1. They compared effectiveness with cost between combined and non-combined treatment
2. They used 1573 adults over the age of 18 with or without radiating symptoms.
3. They were randomly placed into one of the two groups
4. They used the Roland Morris Disability Questionnaire to assess the condition at the 12-month mark.

What Did They Find?

- Overall, scores were "significantly higher in the intervention group than in the control group" at 4 months and at 12 months.

Jeff S. Williams, DC, FIANM

- At the 12-month mark, the combined care model showed an increase in "generic health benefit" AND "cost savings" when compared with the control group.

Wrap It Up

When properly screened and treated, a combined approach to treatment of acute low back pain "will have important implications for the future management of back pain in primary care[12]."

HOW DOES CHIROPRACTIC FIT INTO THE MEDICARE POPULATION?

Medicare is something of an enigma for Doctors of Chiropractic. Here's why: they have decided to reimburse chiropractors at a higher rate than normal as of 2015 so chiropractors are obviously being effective, being efficient, being cost-effective, and over-achieving in general.

However, they still only pay for adjustments.
- No therapy.
- No rehab.
- No exams.
- No x-rays.

Yet, they expect chiropractors to perform some of these when indicated. Now, can one see why a chiropractor would be a bit apprehensive about performing these on Medicare patients when we know that the patient will be forced to pay for them out of pocket?

Chiropractors know full-well that many, if not most, Medicare patients are on a fixed income and have difficulty affording everything we would typically recommend.

Then why not just perform the code and not charge the patient for the service? That is because Medicare was difficult enough to throw in a law that says chiropractors cannot offer any Medicare patient a free service under threat of Federal penalty. It would be viewed as an enticement.

That is a little unfair in my opinion.

WHY THEY DID IT
The authors were interested in how chiropractic compares to the more traditional medical path of care throughout 1 year.

HOW THEY DID IT
- They used 12,170 person-year observations
- They used 5 function measures and 2 measures of self-rated health
- The compared medical vs chiropractic treatment on 1-year changes in regard to function, health, and satisfaction.

WHAT THEY FOUND
- "The unadjusted models show that chiropractic is significantly protective against 1-year decline in activities of daily living, lifting, stooping, walking, self-rated health, and worsening health after 1 year.
- Persons using chiropractic are more satisfied with their follow-up care and with the information provided to them.
- In addition to the protective effects of chiropractic in the unadjusted model, the propensity score results indicate a significant protective effect of chiropractic against decline in reaching."

WRAP UP
Chiropractic showed clear and clinically-significant protective effect against health and ability decline at the 1-year mark among Medicare patients and their conditions of the spine. There are clear indications that patients undergoing chiropractic care also have a higher rate of satisfaction[13].

TREATMENT STUDIES

PREVENTATIVE CHIROPRACTIC CARE – SYSTEMATIC REVIEW

This paper is called "Chiropractic maintenance care – what's new? A systematic review of the literature". It was published in Chiropractic and Manual Therapies and authored by Axen et al[14] in November 2019

Why They Did It
Here's why they did this one: knowing that maintenance care is an age old tradition with chiropractors, and knowing that systematic reviews in '96 and in '08 both found evidence lacking for maintenance care, and then considering Andreas Eklund's Nordic papers on maintenance care (see below), these authors decided to review the newest evidence on the matter.

Wrap Up
Knowledge of chiropractic maintenance care has advanced. There is reasonable consensus among chiropractors on what maintenance care is, how it should be used, and its indications.

Presently, maintenance care can be considered an evidence-based method to perform secondary or tertiary prevention in patients with previous episodes of low back pain who report a good outcome from the initial treatments.

However, these results should not be interpreted as an indication for maintenance care on all patients who receive chiropractic treatment.

THE NORDIC PAPERS ON MAINTENANCE CARE

"The Nordic Maintenance Care program: Effectiveness of chiropractic maintenance care versus symptom-guided treatment for recurrent and persistent low back pain – pragmatic randomized controlled trial" and it was compiled by Andreas Eklund, et. al[15].

Why They Did It

The authors wanted to explore maintenance and preventative treatment in the chiropractic profession. What is the effectiveness for prevention of pain in patients with recurrent or persistent non-specific low back pain?

How They Did It

- 328 patients
- Pragmatic, investigator-blinded. Pragmatic. What does that mean exactly? According to Califf and Sugarman 2015, It means it is *"Designed for the primary purpose of informing decision-makers regarding the comparative balance of benefits, burdens and risks of a biomedical or behavioral health intervention at the individual or population level"* Meaning they are attempting to run a trial to inform decision-makers of responsible guidelines going forward.
- Two arm randomized controlled trial
- Included patients 18-65 w/ non-specific low back pain
- The patients all experienced an early favorable result with chiropractic care.
- After an initial course of treatment ended, the patients were randomized into either a maintenance care group or a control group.
- The control group still received chiropractic care, but on a symptom-related basis.
- The main outcome measured was the number of days with bothersome low back pain during a 1-year period.
- The info was collected weekly through text messaging.

Jeff S. Williams, DC, FIANM

What They Found
- Maintenance care showed a reduction in the number of days per week having low back pain
- During the year-long study, the chiropractic maintenance and preventative treatment group showed 12.8 fewer days.
- The chiropractic maintenance and preventative treatment group received 1.7 more treatments than the symptom-related group.

Wrap It Up
The authors wrap it up by saying, "Maintenance care was more effective than symptom-guided treatment in reducing the total number of days over 52 weeks with bothersome non-specific LBP but it resulted in a higher number of treatments. For selected patients with recurrent or persistent non-specific LBP who respond well to an initial course of chiropractic care, MC should be considered an option for tertiary prevention."

Basically, both groups still underwent chiropractic maintenance and chiropractic preventative treatment. It's like we tell people, stay on a schedule and you'll do well. Wait until you hurt, and the chances are good that you'll spend the same amount getting over that complaint anyway.

This study showed exactly that, except over the course of just one year, the maintenance chiropractic care (preventative chiropractic care) people had 1.7 more visits but suffered pain almost 13 days less.

THE NORDIC PAPERS:
WHICH PATIENTS DO WELL WITH MAINTENANCE CARE?

I welcome another paper by Andreas Eklund on the preventative, maintenance, wellness care.

Eklund's second paper is called "The Nordic Maintenance Care **Program:** Does psychological profile modify the treatment effect of a preventive manual therapy intervention? A secondary analysis of a pragmatic randomized controlled trial" and was published on October 10, 2019[16]. This was a great step forward in validating chiropractic maintenance care.

Why They Did It
The objective was to investigate whether patients in specific psychological sub-groups had different responses to Chiropractic maintenance care regarding the total number of days with bothersome pain and the number of treatments.

How They Did It
- They took data from a two-arm randomized pragmatic multicenter trial
- There was a 12-month follow up
- The follow up was designed to investigate the effectiveness of maintenance care
- Test subjects had recurrent and persistent low back pain
- Patients were randomized to either maintenance care or to symptom-related care
- The primary outcome checked was the total number of days with bothersome low back pain. It was collected weekly for 12 months.
- Total number of subjects was 252

What They Found

- Patients in the dysfunctional subgroup that received MC had fewer days in pain and an equal number of treatments compared to the symptom-related group
- In the adaptive coper subgroup, patients receiving MC had more days with pain and more treatments.
- Patients in the interpersonally distressed subgroup had equal number of days with pain and more treatments with MC

Wrap It Up

Psychological and behavioral characteristics modify the effect of MC and should be considered when recommending long-term preventive management of patients with recurrent and persistent LBP.

What does that mean to us? Well, if we dive into the paper and read the conclusion, we can get a bit more clarity.

They say, if we're going to be recommending chiropractic maintenance care, we need to be making that recommendation to the right kind of patient. Evidently, chiropractic maintenance care isn't effective for everyone.

They say, "Patients who show a favorable response to an initial course of chiropractic care should be considered for chiropractic maintenance care if they report high pain severity, marked interference with everyday life due to pain, high affective distress, low perception of life control and low activity levels at baseline."

I beg for patients like this because I like to be the hero and I know I can help people like this. High pain just means there is nowhere to go but to feel better.

Interference with daily life, high distress, low perception of life control, low levels of activity; those things ALL spell H-E-R-O in my office because we chiropractors can absolutely nail this type of case.

They say that, on the other hand, if a patient reports low pain severity, low interference with everyday life due to pain, low life distress, high activity levels and a high perception of life control, they probably should not be recommended chiropractic maintenance care and should only get symptom-related care. They need to see a chiropractor on an as needed basis basically.

NORDIC PAPERS:
PREVENTATIVE PAPER #3

"The Nordic maintenance care program: maintenance care reduces the number of days with pain in acute episodes and increases the length of pain free periods for dysfunctional patients with recurrent and persistent low back pain – a secondary analysis of a pragmatic randomized controlled trial" by Andreas Eklund et al[17] and published in Chiropractic and Manual Therapies in April 2020.

Why They Did It
Eklund has shown in two previous papers the benefit of treating preventatively, but the benefit varied across psychological subgroups.

The aims of this study were to investigate
1. Pain trajectories around treatments,
2. Recurrence of new episodes of LBP, and
3. Length of consecutive pain-free periods and total number of pain-free weeks, for all study participants as well as for each psychological subgroup.

How They Did It
A secondary analysis of data from a randomized controlled trial of patients seeking chiropractic care for recurrent or persistent LBP used 52 weekly estimates of days with low back pain that limited activity.

What They Found

- Patients receiving maintenance care had flat pain trajectories around each new treatment period and reported fewer days with pain compared to patients receiving the control intervention.
- The entire effect was attributed to the dysfunctional subgroup who reported fewer days with activity limiting pain within each new LBP episode as well as longer total pain-free periods between episodes with a difference of 9.8 weeks compared to the control group.
- There were no differences in the time to/risk of a new episode of LBP in either of the subgroups.

Wrap It Up

Data support the use of MC in a stratified care model targeting dysfunctional patients for MC. For a carefully selected group of patients with recurrent and persistent LBP the clinical course becomes more stable and the number of pain-free weeks between episodes increases when receiving MC.

CHIROPRACTIC RESEARCH AFTER SEVEN LONG YEARS

Dr. Richard Sarnat, MD and Dr. James Winterstein, DC took on a **seven-year study.**

Why They Did It

The question was, "What would happen if there were an unbiased study having to do with chiropractors and led by a medical doctor?" What would it show?

Would all the hearsay and folklore about chiropractic be shown to be true or would chiropractic come out on top?

- The initial study took in stats from 1999 through to 2002.
- The expanded study included stats from 2003-2005.

What They Found

For the entire seven-year period, from 1999 to 2005, patients treating primarily with chiropractors experienced:
- 60% less stays at the hospital
- 62% less outpatient surgical cases
- 85% less pharmaceutical cost
- Higher patient satisfaction

Wrap It Up

Dr. Sarnat was quoted as saying, "I have always believed that the over-utilization of pharmaceuticals and surgery, and the underutilization of more natural healing techniques, such as chiropractic, has been the cause of great suffering. Yet, I had no idea that the magnitude of both clinical improvements and cost effectiveness would approach 50% in both cases.

"Previous studies have shown these types of savings when Chiropractic has been used as a first-line treatment for NMS (neuromusculoskeletal) ailments. But to see this level of effectiveness across the board for literally all types of clinical presentations within a primary care setting is surprising to me, and good news for the rest of the world[18]."

THE USELESSNESS OF GABAPENTIN FOR RADICULAR PAIN

"Anticonvulsants in the Treatment of Low Back Pain and Lumbar Radicular Pain: A Systematic Review and Meta-Analysis" by Enke et. al.[19] published in the Canadian Medical Association Journal in July 2018.

Why They Did It

The use of anticonvulsants (e.g., gabapentin, pregabalin) to treat low back pain has increased substantially in recent years despite limited supporting evidence. We aimed to determine the efficacy and tolerability of anticonvulsants in the treatment of low back pain and lumbar radicular pain compared with placebo.

How They Did It

- A search was conducted in 5 databases for studies comparing an anticonvulsant to placebo in patients with nonspecific low back pain, sciatica, or neurogenic claudication of any duration.
- The outcomes were self-reported pain, disability, and adverse events.
- Risk of bias was assessed using the Physiotherapy Evidence Database (PEDro) scale
- Quality of evidence was assessed using Grading of Recommendations Assessment, Development and Evaluation (GRADE)
- Nine trials compared topiramate, gabapentin or pregabalin to placebo in 859 unique participants.

What They Found

- Fourteen of 15 comparisons found anticonvulsants were not effective to reduce pain or disability in low back pain or lumbar radicular pain.
- For example, there was high-quality evidence of no effect of gabapentinoids versus placebo on chronic low back pain in the short term or for lumbar radicular pain in the immediate term
- This lack of efficacy is accompanied by increased risk of adverse events from use of gabapentinoids, for which the level of evidence is high.

Wrap It Up

"There is moderate- to high-quality evidence that anticonvulsants are ineffective for treatment of low back pain or lumbar radicular pain.

There is high-quality evidence that gabapentinoids have a higher risk of adverse events."

THE UK BEAM STUDY: CHIROPRACTIC & EXERCISE IS THE WAY TO GO FOR BACK PAIN

A widespread study was carried out in the UK for their National Health Service (NHS). It concerned researching the effectiveness of exercise alone, manipulation/mobilization alone, and the two combined for the treatment of back pain.

Why They Did It
The authors wanted to explore the effectiveness of the three options for treatment of back pain for possible recommendations in the National Health Service for the UK primary practitioners.

How They Did It
- This study was a pragmatic randomized trial.
- They used 181 general practices
- 63 community settings in 14 centers in the UK
- 1334 patients were used in the study.
- The Roland-Morris disability questionnaire was used for the Outcome Assessments at the 3-month mark and at the 12-month mark.

What They Found
- All groups improved somewhat over time.
- Exercise helped at the 3-month mark.

- Manipulation was effective at the 3-month mark as well as the 12-month mark.
- Manipulation followed by Exercise was even more effective at both marks.

Wrap It Up

When compared to "best care" practices for general practitioners in the UK's NHS system, Manipulation followed by Exercise was the moderately better overall treatment for back pain[20].

ARE CHIROPRACTORS GREEDY & EXPENSIVE?

One of the misperceptions I hear from time to time is that chiropractors are greedy or that they just want to see how many times they can get a patient in and out of their doors based purely on financial gain. "Once you go to a chiropractor, you have to go the rest of your life." Right?

Let's not beat around the bush here: there most certainly are opportunists in **EVERY** profession in the world. I can be honest and say that chiropractic is no exception.

However, in general, people are good by nature and chiropractors are no exception. Truly, most chiropractors got into business to help people. No other reason. Just to help.

Before we dive into the research, ask yourself a simple question, "If my primary sent me to a physical therapist, would they just see me once and then tell me to call if it keeps bothering me?" If you've had any experience with physical therapy, you already know the answer to that question.

Of course not!

You'll be treated on a steady and consistent basis for a specific amount of time, because any change in the body, or substantial healing, takes time and consistency. In addition, building any significant durability to avoid future worsening of the original injury is something that takes work. This is mostly common sense.

That being said, let's dive in. The Manga Report is an old chiropractic stand-by. This report has been around for some time now. Since 1993 to be exact.

Why They Did It
To assess the effectiveness in terms of physical recovery or pain alleviation as well as the cost-effectiveness of chiropractic in regard to treating low back pain.

How They Did It
The Ontario Ministry of Health-commissioned study was a comprehensive review of all of the published literature on low back pain.

What They Found
What they found is astounding:
- They found an overwhelming amount of evidence showing the effectiveness of chiropractic in the treatment of low back pain and complaint.
- They also found that it is more cost-effective than traditional medical treatment and management.
- They found that many of the traditional medical therapies used in low back pain are considered questionable in validity, and although some are very safe, some can lead to other problems for the patient.
- There are no case controlled studies that even hint that chiropractic is not safe for the treatment of low back pain. They showed that chiropractic is clearly more cost-effective and there would be highly significant savings if more low back pain management was controlled by chiropractors rather than medical physicians.

- The study stated that chiropractic services should be fully insured.
- The study stated that services should be fully integrated into the overall healthcare system due to the high cost of low back pain and the cost-effectiveness and physical effectiveness of chiropractic.
- They also stated that a good case could be made for making chiropractors the entry point into the healthcare system for musculoskeletal complaints that presented to hospitals.

Wrap It Up

Chiropractic should be the treatment of choice for low back pain, even excluding traditional medical care altogether[21]!

ACUPUNCTURE FOR CHRONIC PAIN

"Acupuncture for Chronic Pain: Update of an Individual Patient Data Meta-Analysis" by Vickers et. al[22] published in Journal of Pain in May of 2018.

Why They Did It

Despite wide use in clinical practice, acupuncture remains a controversial treatment for chronic pain. Our objective was to update an individual patient data meta-analysis to determine the effect size of acupuncture for 4 chronic pain conditions

How They Did It
- They searched MEDLINE and the Cochrane Central Registry of Controlled Trials randomized trials published up until December 31, 2015.
- They included randomized trials of acupuncture needling versus either sham acupuncture or no acupuncture control for nonspecific musculoskeletal pain, osteoarthritis, chronic headache, or shoulder pain.

- Trials were only included if allocation concealment was unambiguously determined to be adequate.
- Raw data were obtained from study authors and entered in an individual patient data meta-analysis.
- The main outcome measures were pain and function.
- An additional 13 trials were identified, with data received for a total of 20,827 patients from 39 trials

What They Found
- Acupuncture was superior to sham as well as to no acupuncture control for each pain condition
- They also found clear evidence that the effects of acupuncture persist over time with only a small decrease, approximately 15%, in treatment effect at 1 year

Wrap It Up
The authors wrap it up by concluding, "Acupuncture is effective for the treatment of chronic pain, with treatment effects persisting over time. Although factors in addition to the specific effects of needling at correct acupuncture point locations are important contributors to the treatment effect, decreases in pain after acupuncture cannot be explained solely in terms of placebo effects"

PIONEERING RESEARCH INTO CHRONIC LOW BACK PAIN TREATMENT

Why They Did It
The authors of this paper wanted to compare hospital outpatient treatment with chiropractic treatment and their efficacy in treating long-term low back pain of mechanical origin.

How They Did It
- The study was a randomized controlled trial.
- The setting was in chiropractic clinics as well as in hospital outpatient clinics.

- 741 patients were used for the study.
- The patients ranged in age from 18-65
- The patients had to have been free of any treatment for the previous month.
- The Outcome Assessment was via the Oswestry pain disability questionnaire, the straight leg raising test, and in lumbar flexion.

What They Found
- Chiropractic was found to be superior over hospital outpatient management.
- Mostly for chronic or severe back pain.

Wrap It Up
"For patients with low back pain in whom manipulation is not contraindicated chiropractic almost certainly confers worthwhile, long term benefit in comparison with hospital outpatient management. The benefit is seen mainly in those with chronic or severe pain[23]."

CHIROPRACTIC WELLNESS: IS THERE ANY PROOF THAT IT WORKS?

There has been a lot of research coming out in recent years thanks to Palmer College in Davenport, Iowa, National Health Interview Survey, and Gallup Poll. I am happy to share you that the news is all good for Chiropractic!

The National Health Interview Survey recently did an updated survey called "Wellness-related Use of Common Complementary Health Approaches Among Adults: The United States, 2012."

The results of this survey were published by the University of Maryland School of Medicine's Center for Integrative Medicine. Again, the results were all good. Over 50% of the people surveyed said that they use chiropractic treatment for wellness.

More than 65% said that they use chiropractic to treat specific health conditions. Also in 2015 Gallup did a poll regarding Americans' perceptions of chiropractic. The poll showed that:

- Over 50% of American adults viewed chiropractors positively
- Chiropractors are effective in the treatment of back and neck pain.
- 31% of chiropractic patients enjoy going to the chiropractor regularly even in the absence of pain.
- 22% of American adults seek a chiropractor's advice regarding general health and wellness.

In addition, a four-year long study called, "Clinical and Cost Outcomes of An Integrative Medicine IPA," was published in the Journal of Manipulative and Physiological Therapeutics. Once again, chiropractic was the bright point. The study showed the chiropractic patients that use chiropractic and other integrative alternatives experienced a significant amount of improved wellness over those that did not use these services.

- These patients saw 43% fewer hospital admissions
- They had 58.4% fewer days spent in the hospital
- 43.2% fewer surgeries and procedures
- Their pharmaceutical costs went down by 51.8%

Chiropractors may be known to the layperson as "back crackers" or "bone poppers," however chiropractic training includes 4,620 hours of schooling including nutrition, physiology, rehabilitation, the exact same basic sciences as medical schools, and many tons of wellness topics. One would be correct in considering chiropractors to be experts in the wellness arena.

When one is even mildly knowledgeable of the research, there is little doubt left that chiropractic works in just about every aspect of the healthcare field including overall wellness[24].

CHIROPRACTIC MORE COST-EFFECTIVE AND MORE EFFECTIVE OVERALL THAN GENERAL PRACTITIONER

Why They Did It

The authors of this paper wished to perform a review of trial-based economic evaluations that have been performed for manual therapy in comparison to other treatment protocols used for treatment of musculoskeletal complaints.

How They Did It
- The authors performed a comprehensive literature search of commonly used research databases for all subjects relative to this subject.
- 25 publications were included.
- The studies included cost-effectiveness for manual therapies compared to other forms of treatment for pain.

What They Found
- Manual therapy techniques such as chiropractic mobilization were more cost effective than visiting a general practitioner.
- Specifically, chiropractic treatment was less costly and was found to be more effective than physiotherapy/physical therapy and visiting a general practitioner's medical office when treating neck pain.

Wrap It Up

Although improvement in our knowledge of manual therapies is warranted, this paper demonstrates that chiropractic is more cost-effective and more effective in general for low back pain & shoulder disability than usual medical practitioner care and physical therapy/physiotherapy[25].

CHRONIC SPINAL PAIN AND CHIROPRACTIC. SIGNIFICANT RESULTS

Why Did They Do It?

The authors wanted to test and compare effectiveness of chiropractic manipulation in chronic spinal pain complaints. They used several different protocols including needle acupuncture, non-steroidal anti-inflammatory medication, and/or chiropractic manipulation.

How Did They Do It?

- 77 patients randomly assigned to receive one of the treatment protocols
- 30 days of treatments
- Symptoms and changes were assessed through Outcome Assessment questionnaires (Oswestry Back Pain Disability Index, Neck Disability Index, and VAS scales).
- What Did They Find?
- After 30 days, spinal manipulation was the only intervention to achieve statistically significant improvement.
- Chiropractic care = 30.7% reduction in Oswestry scores, 25% reduction in neck disability scores.
- VAS scores were 50% less for low back pain, 46% less for upper back pain, and 33% less for neck pain.

Wrap It Up

Chiropractic is the treatment of choice in chronic spinal pain (low back, upper back, neck pain). It is certainly the treatment of choice compared to acupuncture and anti-inflammatory medication[26].

MANUAL THERAPY MORE EFFECTIVE, LESS EXPENSIVE

This research goes a long way toward showing the **cost-effectiveness** and the **overall effectiveness** of manual therapy/spinal mobilization when compared to traditional medical treatment or physiotherapy/physical therapy alone.

Why They Did It
The authors wanted to evaluate, contrast, and compare effectiveness of manual therapy to physiotherapy/physical therapy and to care by a general medical practitioner in regard to neck pain specifically.

How They Did It
- This was an economic evaluation in addition to a randomized controlled trial.
- 183 Participants with neck pain for 2 weeks in duration
- 42 General medical practitioners
- The patients were randomly treated with manual therapy/spinal mobilization, physiotherapy/physical therapy, or general practitioner protocols
- Clinical results were based on perceived recovery, intensity of pain, functional disability, and quality of life changes.
- Cost-efficiency was determined by the patients' keeping a log of costs for one year.

What They Found
Manual therapy/spinal mobilization shown to be faster in regard to improvement than BOTH physiotherapy/physical therapy and general practitioner protocols for up to 26 weeks.

The cost of manual therapy/spinal mobilization therapy was roughly 1/3 the cost of physiotherapy/physical therapy and general practitioner protocols.

Manual therapy/spinal mobilization was proven through research to be significantly more effective and cost less in the treatment of neck pain when compared to physiotherapy/physical therapy and general practitioners[27].

WHY NERVE ROOT INJECTION DESERVE MORE CONSIDERATION

In this article we compare shots in the neck or cervical region to spinal manipulative therapy, which is also known as chiropractic adjustment.

In other articles, I have highlighted the lack of evidence for the use of the epidural spinal injections and the lack of effectiveness beyond short-term reduction of inflammation. Epidural spinal injections have shown no benefit at all beyond some short-term pain and inflammation reduction and zero usefulness in regard to long-term disability or the eventual need for surgery. Zero.

A paper by Nancy Epstein in 2013 and published in Surgical Neurology International stated, "Although not approved by the Food and Drug Administration (FDA), injections are being performed with an increased frequency (160%), are typically short-acting and ineffective over the longer-term, while exposing patients to major risks/complications."

In addition to that information, there is research showing that each subsequent epidural spinal injection puts the patient at a 26% greater risk of spinal fracture down the road. My question is, "Why on Earth are people getting these injections at such an alarming rate when the research is taken into account?"

The only logical answer is that the research isn't being considered at all. One would think these injections would be on the decline. However, despite the research showing their ineffectiveness, the popularity of injections has only increased. Don't take my word for it. Consumer Reports said, "Controversy surrounds these injections, and use has increased dramatically in recent years, along with escalating costs." They went on to add, "Some experts believe that their growth reflects—in part—the rising prevalence of lower-back pain. But others suspect it's driven by financial incentives."

"Our analysis of the evidence, based on a recent report by the American Society of Health-System Pharmacists and several published reviews and treatment guidelines, suggests that while the shots might have limited value by providing short-term relief to some people, in most cases people should try other measures first."

With all factors considered, let's look at this week's research comparing injections to chiropractic adjustments for neck pain.

Why They Did It
The authors wanted to attempt to measure the overall outcomes regarding pain, improvement, and costs of cervical (neck) root injection blocks vs. chiropractic spinal manipulative therapy.

How They Did It
- The study included 104 participants.
- Each had a disc herniation that was confirmed by MRI.
- 52 underwent treatment via the nerve root block.
- 52 underwent chiropractic spinal manipulative therapy.
- Baseline pain scores were collected on each individual using the numerical rating scale (NRS).
- The NRS was also taken three months after the end of treatment for improvement comparison.
- Improvement was measured with the Patient Global Impression of Change scale.

What They Found

- 86.5% of participants in the chiropractic spinal manipulative therapy group showed significant improvement.
- Only 49% of the nerve root block group reported improvement.

Wrap It Up

"Subacute/chronic patients treated with SMT were significantly more likely to report relevant "improvement" compared with CNRI patients. There was no difference in outcomes when comparing acute patients only."

As a result, the next time anyone tells you to get nerve blocks or an epidural injection for pain as a result of a herniated disc, consider this information and consider getting a second opinion from an evidence-based, patient-centered chiropractor before undergoing a mostly useless and potentially dangerous treatment protocol[28].

SHOULD YOU START CARE WITH A CHIROPRACTOR OR A MEDICAL DOCTOR?

Before getting into the research for this paper, I wanted to provide a story about one man who was a patient of mine for years. One day, he shared with me the fact that I gave him the ability to get out of the house and got him active with his grandkids and active in his job again. His exact words were, "You saved my life."

I didn't understand how that could be true, so he explained what he meant. He recalled that when he first came to see me, he couldn't even roll over and had been that way for years. He couldn't sit up on his own. He was in terrible condition physically.

With some work, not only were we able to get him active and playing games like washers and horseshoes in his back yard, but he also got inspired to quit smoking! This patient and I became good friends over the years.

Unfortunately, he passed on a few years ago but he told me I gave him his life back. I can't tell you how special something like that is to me.

When I think about whether you should start care with a chiropractor or a medical doctor, I think about that patient. I think about how he had been to his primary care doctor for years and he had never addressed simple issues like movement and mobilization. I also thought about how we were able to help make his remaining time on Earth quality years spent with his family rather than years spent lying in bed in pain, smoking cigarettes, and unable to move.

Other than pills and shots, which can have harmful side effects, I've seen nothing as effective for treating neuromusculoskeletal complaints such as back pain, neck pain, headaches, sciatica, overall stiffness, or disc complaints.

Here's a recent study that was published in the Journal of Manipulative and Physiological Therapeutics in 2015.

Why They Did It:
The authors of the paper wanted to see the difference in patient satisfaction and healthcare costs for conditions such as spinal pain, hip, and shoulder pain in patients that started their care with a medical doctor compared with those that started their care with a doctor of chiropractic.

How They Did It:
- A questionnaire was completed by the patients in the study.
- Their healthcare costs were then determined.
- 403 patients were seen first by a medical doctor.
- 316 were seen first by a chiropractor.

- The patients attending the medical doctor first had significantly less improvement in pain level and were significantly less satisfied with their treatment outcome and care received.

Wrap Up

There was significantly greater satisfaction and lower cost when a patient initiated care with a chiropractor rather than a medical doctor for musculoskeletal conditions of the spine, hip, and shoulder. [29].

CHIROPRACTIC EFFECTIVE FOR HEADACHES AND MIGRAINES

I can't tell you how many patients come in to see chiropractors for headaches. I have seen them range from life-long headaches & migraines all the way to, "I woke up this morning with a headache."

I have had different levels of success with headaches. My most memorable success was a patient that had headaches her entire life. She had nuclear bone scans. She had injections in the back of her head. She had MRI's that came back normal. Yet, she continued to be plagued by headaches daily.

After initializing treatment, it literally took only two weeks and she stopped having headaches. **That was years ago, and she still does not suffer from headaches!**

We DO, from time to time, run into a headache that won't respond to treatment, but that is rare and probably includes only 10%-15% of headache patients. **Chiropractic just works with headaches.** Here's more proof!

Why They Did It:
Since chronic headaches have a substantial socioeconomic impact, the authors/researchers were interested in what part spinal manipulative therapy (SMT) could play in helping the situation.

How They Did It:
- Randomized clinical trials
- The trials had to include, at the least, one patient-related outcome measure
- They used a search of MEDLINE and EMBASE databases to find trials that fit the protocol
- They used all data from Cumulative Index of Nursing and Allied Health Literature
- They used the Chiropractic Research Archives Collection,
- They used the Manual, Alternative, and Natural Therapies Information System
- Nine trials involving 683 patients

What They Found
- Moderate evidence that SMT has significantly more effectiveness than massage in cervicogenic headaches.
- SMT has effects comparable to common prescription medications for tension and migraine headaches.

Wrap It Up
More studies need to be conducted over longer periods of time but, with these studies being randomized clinical trials, the evidence is dependable and shows chiropractic to be very effective for headaches and migraines while avoiding medication and their associated side effects[30].

HOW RESEARCH MAY CHANGE HOW WE ALL VIEW LOW BACK DISC TREATMENT

At this point in research, it is basic common knowledge, even among chiropractic detractors, that chiropractic manipulation is significantly effective for low back pain.

However, not as much evidence exists regarding manipulative treatment for complaints originating from lumbar disc herniation. We chiropractors see the effectiveness daily, but backing research is always very satisfying.

Why They Did It
The authors in this paper were curious as to the safety and effectiveness of mobilization/manipulation of a lumbar disc herniation.

How They Did It
- The authors extracted the pertinent information from commonly used research databases such as PubMed, OVID, Cochrane Library, CBM, CNKI, and VIP.
- 832 papers on the topic (lumbar disc herniations) were extracted for the study.
- 8 of the papers met the criteria for the study and were subsequently used.
- There were 911 low back disc herniation patients within the qualifying 8 articles.
- The data was processed using the Cochrane systematic review process.

What They Found
The cure rate for patients undergoing chiropractic manipulative treatment was greater than with other treatment methods, which included acupuncture, traction, thermotherapy, etc.

Jeff S. Williams, DC, FIANM

"This study shows that manipulative treatment on lumbar disc herniation is safe, effective, and both cure rate and the effective rate is better than other therapies." However, the authors also admit that higher quality evidence needs to be collected for a higher level of validation[31].

THE DARK SECRET OF EPIDURAL STEROID INJECTIONS

I see people weekly who are considering epidural steroid injections. Patients consider this procedure for several reasons. The most common reasons are conditions such as musculoskeletal pain (especially in the low back and neck), nerve pain or radiculopathy, and/or spinal stenosis.

I stress to these patients that there is solid research showing that these injections are only good for short-term use and only in a certain percentage of people. When they do work, they usually have to be repeated since they commonly do not last very long. This makes sense, because the injections are only treating the inflammation caused by the irritated disc or nerve.

Essentially, it's like taking the battery out of the smoke alarm, but the fire is still raging.

The national pain report tells us that nearly 9,000,000 spinal injections are performed annually in the United States. Some of the side effects and drawbacks of the epidural steroid injections are as follows:
- Arachnoiditis, which is an inflammation and infection in the membrane around the spinal cord.
- Increased risk of spinal fractures due to bone deterioration.
- Nerve damage due to the needle contacting the nerves

- Bleeding due to an underlying disorder
- Dural puncture
- Increased pain rather than decreased pain
- Headaches
- Sleeplessness or fever
- Stomach ulcers
- Cataracts

Patients accept all this risk for a very short-term solution that works less than 50% of the time and costs over $2000 per injection. It makes absolutely zero sense outside of an emergency.

Considering this information, let's get to the research. After you read it, you may wonder why the medical world continues to chastise chiropractors for treating back pain successfully through natural remedies.

Why They Did It
The use of epidural steroid injections is on the rise every year. The authors of this paper wanted to review the evidence regarding the pros and cons of epidural steroid injections used in adults suffering from low back pain that radiated and in adults with spinal stenosis.

How They Did It
- They used common and standard data sources such as Ovid MEDLINE (through May 2015), Cochrane Central Register of Controlled Trials, Cochrane Database of Systematic Reviews, prior systematic reviews, and reference lists.
- From these databases they selected trials versus placebo interventions or studies comparing epidural injection techniques, corticosteroids, or different doses.

What They Found
- 30 placebo trials studied injections used for radiculopathy
- Eight studies looked at effectiveness for spinal stenosis.

- When treating radiculopathy, injections showed greater immediate reduction in pain, function, and short-term surgery risk.
- The effects were below the predetermined clinically important threshold
- There were no long-term benefits whatsoever.
- Injections had ZERO effects for spinal stenosis.

Wrap It Up

Although steroid injections for radiculopathy showed some short-term relief in pain and short-term increase in function, the benefits seen in the patients were small and short-term only. There was no effect long-term and no effect on whether or not the person had surgery eventually. The evidence in this paper suggested there was no effectiveness at all for the treatment of spinal stenosis[32].

WHY ARE DOCTORS STILL PRESCRIBING EPIDURAL STEROID INJECTIONS?

Why They Did It

Considering the frequency with which epidural spinal injections are being used to control low back pain and radiating, shooting pain into legs, the authors felt it necessary to review the current evidence for the benefits and harms of these injections. This particularly concerned injections in the epidural space, the facet joints, and the sacroiliac regions.

How They Did It

The researcher used the following sources:
- Systematic review of searches through July 2008
- Electronic databases from January 2008 through October 2014
- Reference lists
- Clinical trials registries

- They selected randomized trials of patients having lumbosacral radiating pain, spinal stenosis, pain that did not run into the leg(s), or more chronic back pain after a surgery.
- These research abstracts compared how effective the injections were vs. a placebo.

What They Found
- In regard to radiculopathy (Shooting pain into a leg or both legs) the only improvement noted was for pain at the immediate follow-up, improvement in function at immediate follow-up, and decreased risk of surgery at immediate follow-up.
- The effects were small and did not meet the requirement for them to be minimally important.
- There was no benefit in long-term follow-up.
- In regard to the injection itself, it did not seem to matter what technique was used.
- In regard to spinal stenosis, there was limited evidence for any effectiveness and no differences in pain, function, or likelihood of surgery.
- In regard to the facet joint, there was no clear effectiveness.

Wrap It Up
For radiating pain/symptoms, epidural corticosteroid injections had only immediate effectiveness in function, pain, and likelihood of surgery. However, the benefits were small, un-sustained, and having no effect at all on long-term risk of surgery.

What Are You Not Being Told About Spinal Injections?

Why They Did It
The purpose of this study was to compare the outcomes of overall improvement, pain reduction, and cost effectiveness in paired, similar patients with characteristic MRI-confirmed disc herniations in the neck region. The patients were treated with either chiropractic mobilization or injections in the cervical region.

How They Did It
- The study consisted of 104 patients
- All had herniated discs in the neck region that were confirmed through MRIs.
- 52 patients were treated with injections to the neck region.
- 52 patients treated with chiropractic spinal mobilization.
- The Numeric Ratings Scale was used to assess pain levels at baseline, at 3 months after treatment.
- Overall "improvement" was assessed using the Patient Global Impression of Change Scale also at the three-month mark.
- The only responses on the scale that were accepted as an improvement were "much better" or "better."
- NRS numbers were compared at baseline and at the 3-month measuring.

What They Found
- "Improvement" was reported in 86.5% of the patients that underwent chiropractic spinal manipulative treatment.
- Only 49.0% of patients that received injections reported improvement.
- Significantly more patients undergoing injections were in the subacute/chronic category (77%) compared with those patients that were in the spinal manipulative chiropractic treatment group (46%).

Wrap It Up
Subacute/chronic patients treated with SMT were much more likely to report improvement than were those who had injections. For acute cases there was no difference.

Since chiropractic treatment was superior to spinal injections in subacute/chronic patients, since several research papers have shown the injections to be strictly short-term in nature with zero long-term effect, since they are far more expensive than chiropractic treatment, and since there was no proven superior effect in the acute patients,[28] chiropractic is the better choice.

WHY CHIROPRACTIC IS
THE SECRET WEAPON FOR BACK & NECK PAIN

Regardless of the evidence and research, including randomized controlled trials, that are out there in support of chiropractic, manual therapies, and spinal mobilization, there are those who continue to disparage the profession rather than educate themselves on its efficacy.

I believe it is true that we have outliers in every industry, including the chiropractic profession. Most people are sensible and understand that there are outlier plumbers that will take advantage of a person just because they are in the position to do so. There are mechanics changing out and charging for perfectly good automotive parts, and surgeons doing questionable or unnecessary surgery.

There are insurance salesmen that will sell you insurance coverage they know you do not really need. In my profession, there are chiropractors that will make claims they should not make and will treat you when it will not necessarily make much difference to your current or future health at all.

I think it is understandable that outliers exist and avoiding them is just part of navigating our way through life. There is even a quote for it. It goes like this, "Fool me once, shame on you. Fool me twice, shame on me."

But it seems that outliers get more attention in the chiropractic profession than do the highly educated and highly professional practitioners that are getting people well every single day. Too often the loud minority gets the attention. That is, for obvious reasons, highly frustrating.

It is only through continual and consistent sharing of research and evidence that the chiropractic profession will change and eventually overcome this situation. I have faith that solid research and evidence can only be ignored for a specific amount of time.

With that in mind, here is some research showing effectiveness of spinal manipulative therapy and/or mobilization for low back and neck pain.

Why They Did It
As stated above, the authors felt there were a multitude of randomized clinical trials, reviews, and national clinical guidelines regarding chiropractic for low back and neck pain, but there still remained some controversy as to its effectiveness among some in the medical field. They wanted to step back and review all the information, only accept valuable papers on the topic, and generate a solid opinion on chiropractic effectiveness for treating low back and neck pain.

How They Did It
- They chose papers on randomized trials from around the world through computerized databases.
- They used two independent reviewers to check the quality of the papers using guidelines laid out before starting the project.
- 69 randomized clinical trials were reviewed.
- Only 43 ultimately met the predetermined criteria and were accepted for the review.

What They Found
- There is moderate evidence that chiropractic has more effectiveness for short-term pain relief than does mobilization and limited evidence of faster recovery over physical therapy.
- For chronic low back pain, there is moderate evidence that spinal manipulative therapy has an effect equal to prescription non-steroidal anti-inflammatory drugs. Also, spinal manipulation and mobilization show effectiveness in

short-term relief over that of a primary practitioner as well as superiority in the long term when compared to physical therapy.

- There is moderate to limited evidence showing that Chiropractic is superior to physical therapy in long-term and short-term treatment of low back pain and neck pain.
- For a mix of short- and long-term pain, chiropractic was either similar or superior to McKenzie exercises, medical treatment, or physical therapy.

Wrap It Up

The authors concluded that "recommendations can be made with confidence regarding the use of spinal manipulative therapy and/or mobilization as a viable option for the treatment of both low back pain and neck pain[33]."

ARE YOU SPENDING TOO MUCH ON THAT NECK PAIN?

This paper shows that it makes more financial sense to seek out a chiropractor for neuromusculoskeletal issues before consulting our medical counterparts.

This article is from 2016.

Why They Did It

The authors on the study wanted to compare how services were used and charged in the healthcare field by doctors of chiropractic and medical doctors.

How They Did It

- They used data from 2000 to 2009 from North Carolina State Health Plan for Teachers and State Employees (NCSHP).
- They used diagnostic codes for uncomplicated neck pain as well as complicated neck pain.

Jeff S. Williams, DC, FIANM

- Single providers that did not refer their patients to others racked up the least in charges on average for both uncomplicated neck pain as well as complicated pain.
- When care did not include referrals, medical doctor care with physical therapy was generally less expensive than medical care and chiropractic care combined.
- But, when treatment protocols included referral providers, medical doctor care, and physical therapist care it was more expensive on the average than medical care combined with chiropractic care for either condition.
- Charges for chiropractic patients in the middle quintiles of risk had lower bills with or without medical care or referral care to other providers.

Wrap It Up

Chiropractic care alone OR chiropractic care in combination with medical care had significantly fewer charges for uncomplicated neck pain or complicated neck pain when compared to the medical care with or without physical therapy care[34].

ISN'T GOING TO THE CHIROPRACTOR RISKY?

Although the plight of the chiropractor has improved over the last 5-10 years, it is still not rare to hear things like, "I wouldn't go to a chiropractor. They'll twist your head off." Or something along the lines of, "My family doctor told me to never let a chiropractor touch my neck."

As you may imagine, as a chiropractor, I hear this sort of talk (and worse) on a regular basis. It can admittedly be discouraging. It is key for a chiropractor to have a short memory on things like this and to develop more confidence in themselves as they watch their patients make miraculous progress over time.

The publication date of this paper was February 15, 2015 in Spine Journal. Spine Journal sounds a bit like a chiropractic publication, but it is not. It is for neurologists, orthopedic surgeons, and everyone else concerned with issues of the spine.

Why They Did It

The researchers felt there was inadequate study into the risk of physical injury from spinal manipulation in older folks (a population at increased risk of any sort of injury) following visits to a doctor of chiropractic vs. a visit to their primary care physician.

How They Did It

- Medicare data was analyzed on patients aged 66-99
- All patients had a visit in 2007 for a neuromusculoskeletal complaint.
- Using standardized testing, the patients were evaluated within 7 days.
- They compared those treated by a doctor of chiropractic against those evaluated by a primary care physician.

What They Found

- The risk for injury in the chiropractic group was lower than that of the primary care group.
- The cumulative probability of injury in the primary care physician group was 153 per 100,000 subjects.
- The cumulative probability of injury in the chiropractic group was 40 injuries per 100,000 subjects.

Wrap It Up

"Among Medicare beneficiaries aged 66-99 with an office visit risk for a neuromusculoskeletal problem, risk of injury to the head, neck, or trunk within 7 days was 76% lower among subjects with a chiropractic office visit than among those who saw a primary care physician[35]

CHIROPRACTIC VS. AMITRIPTYLINE FOR MIGRAINES GRUDGE MATCH

It has been my experience that most people identify chiropractors with back and neck pain but not necessarily headaches or migraines. However, more and more information is coming to light regarding the effectiveness of spinal manipulative therapy for headaches and migraines.

Why They Did It
They estimate that around 11 million Americans have moderate to severe disability from migraines. The authors wanted to get a closer reading on what effectiveness spinal manipulation has on migraine headaches.

How They Did It
- 218 Randomized patients pre-diagnosed with migraines
- Measure efficacy of spinal manipulation
- Measured efficacy of amitriptyline
- Measured efficacy of treatment that combines both manipulation AND amitriptyline

What They Found
- Clinically important improvement observed with the patients undergoing spinal manipulation alone (40%)
- Improvement under amitriptyline (49%)
- Improvement in the group undergoing both treatments. (41%)
- But, upon post-treatment evaluation, A FAR HIGHER AMOUNT OF MIGRAINE PATIENTS THAT UNDERWENT SPINAL MANIPULATION ALONE HAD REDUCTION ON THEIR HEADACHE DISABILITY INDEX SCORES THAN IN THE OTHER TWO GROUPS.

Wrap It Up

Since the study proved that Chiropractic was equal in effectiveness to a an established medical treatment (amitriptyline), then Chiropractic should be considered the reasonable option in complaints such as these[36].

WHAT RESEARCH SAYS ABOUT CHRONIC LOW BACK PAIN

Why They Did It

With chronic back pain so prevalent in our society, its significance cannot be overstated. The authors felt it necessary to attempt to better understand all aspects of low back pain, treatment, and outcomes.

How They Did It

The authors examined the following areas to determine use and effectiveness.

- Imaging
- Opioid Use
- Spinal Injections
- Spinal Surgery

What They Found

- 629% increase Medicare expenditures on epidural spinal injections
- 423% increase for opioids due to back pain
- 307% increase in low back MRIs for beneficiaries of Medicare
- 220% increase in spinal fusion surgeries
- No improvement in patient outcomes and/or disability rates

Wrap It Up

Prescribing yet more imaging, opioids, injections, and operations is not likely to improve outcomes for patients with chronic back pain. We must re- think chronic back pain at fundamental levels. Our understanding of chronic back pain mechanisms remains rudimentary, including our knowledge of spinal biology, central nervous system processing, genetic factors, and psychosocial and environmental influences. Greater investment is needed in this basic science research.

Clinicians may often be applying an acute care model to a chronic condition. There are no "magic bullets" for chronic back pain, and expecting a cure from a drug, injection, or operation is generally wishful thinking[37].

ACUTE & CHRONIC LOW BACK PAIN TREATMENT BY PRIMARY CARE & BY CHIROPRACTIC

Chiropractic and spinal mobilization are becoming more and more accepted by the medical community in the treatment of acute and chronic low back pain. There is even less push-back from the biggest chiropractic detractors in the world when it comes to chiropractic treatment for low back pain specifically. That is how we know the message is truly getting out.

Here's one more example of why there is more and more acceptance among our medical counterparts for chiropractic low back pain treatment.

Why They Did It

The authors wanted to conduct a longer-term study to evaluate low back pain patients 4 years after primary care or chiropractic care.

How They Did It
- It was a prospective, nonrandomized, practice-based study.
- 51 Chiropractic clinics & 60 chiropractors participated
- 14 general practice clinics and 111 general practitioners participated
- 2870 low back pain patients of acute and chronic duration.
- Outcomes were performed using the visual analogue (VAS) scale and Oswestry Questionnaire.
- Outcomes measured at the beginning to establish the baseline and them at 8 different time points up to the 48-month follow-up.

What They Found
- Most of the improvements in the patients were seen at the 3-month point through the 1-year mark, while the more acute patients had relief at all measured time points.
- There was a clinically significant advantage in the short-term for chiropractic patients suffering from chronic pain.
- At the 1-year mark, the acute and chronic patients all had better improvement with chiropractic.
- Chiropractic also beat out primary care for low back pain with associated leg pain below the knee.

Wrap It Up

"Study findings were consistent with systematic reviews of the efficacy of spinal manipulation for pain and disability in acute and chronic LBP. Patient choice and interdisciplinary referral should be prime considerations by physicians, policymakers, and third-party payers in identifying health services for patients with LBP[38]."

COMPARISON OF COMBINED APPROACH TO ACUTE LOW BACK PAIN – 2011

This study was held in the UK in 2011. The study makes mention of "stratified" primary care management which refers to uses of alternative treatment such as manual therapy. So, if when reading this paper, it is appropriate to replace the word "stratified" with alternative treatments or manual therapy.

Why Did They Do It?
The authors were well-aware that back pain remains a significant challenge for primary practitioners to treat and manage. They were also aware of the fact that co-management of back pain among primary practitioners and alternative therapies had yet to be tested.

How They Did It.
- They compared effectiveness with cost between combined treatment and non-combined.
- Included 1573 adults over the age of 18 with or without radiating symptoms.
- Patients were randomly placed into one of the two groups
- They used the Roland Morris Disability Questionnaire to assess the condition at the 12-month mark.

What Did They Find?
- Overall, the scores were "significantly higher in the intervention group than in the control group" at 4 months and at 12 months.
- At the 12-month mark, the combined care model showed an increase in "generic health benefit" AND "cost savings" when compared with the control group.

Wrap It Up
When properly screened and treated, a combined approach to treatment of acute low back pain "will have important implications for the future management of back pain in primary care[12]."

HOW DOES CHIROPRACTIC FIT INTO THE MEDICARE POPULATION?

Medicare is something of an enigma for doctors of chiropractic. Here's why: they have decided to reimburse chiropractors at a higher rate than normal as of 2015, so we're obviously being effective, being efficient, being cost-effective, and over-achieving in general. However, they still only pay for adjustments.

- No therapy.
- No rehab.
- No exams.
- No x-rays.

Yet, they expect chiropractors to perform some of these when indicated. Now, can you see why a chiropractor would be a bit apprehensive about performing these on Medicare patients when we know that the patient will be forced to pay for them out of pocket? We chiropractors know full well that many, if not most, Medicare patients are on a fixed income and have a difficult time affording such care.

Then why not just perform the code and not charge the patient for the service? That would be because Medicare was difficult enough to throw in a law that says chiropractors cannot offer any Medicare patient a free service under threat of federal penalty. It would be viewed as an inducement.

Why They Did It
The authors were interested in how chiropractic compares to the more traditional medical path of care throughout 1 year.

How They Did It
- They used 12,170 person-year observations
- They used 5 function measures and 2 measures of self-rated health

- The compared medical vs chiropractic treatment on 1-year changes in function, health, and satisfaction.

What They Found
- "The unadjusted models show that chiropractic is significantly protective against 1-year decline in activities of daily living, lifting, stooping, walking, self-rated health, and worsening health after 1 year.
- Persons using chiropractic are more satisfied with their follow-up care and with the information provided to them.
- In addition to the protective effects of chiropractic in the unadjusted model, the propensity score results indicate a significant protective effect of chiropractic against decline in reaching."

Wrap It Up
Chiropractic showed clear and clinically significant protective effect against health and ability decline at the 1-year mark among Medicare patients and their conditions of the spine. There are also clear indications that patients undergoing chiropractic care have a higher rate of satisfaction[13].

SURGERY FOR LOW BACK PAIN: REVIEW OF EVIDENCE

Why They Did It
The researchers wanted to update their understanding of the benefits, as well as the harmful effects, of surgery in the cases of non-radiating (no pain into the leg) back pain as well as surgery in patients with common degeneration, and with radiating pain (pain into the leg) due to a herniated disc. They also wanted to update the understanding on surgery for pain due to stenosis of the spine. Spinal surgery is very common these days, but it's still unclear as far as when, where, and why it's being done.

How They Did It
- The researchers used databases called Ovid MEDLINE and Cochrane to search the research abstracts having to do with their study. They took randomized controlled trials and reviews.
- They used 2 independent reviewers.
- They followed specific rules and guidelines in their review of the literature.

What They Found
- In non-radicular low back pain with degeneration, there was fair evidence showing vertebrae fusion to be no better than intensive rehab but slightly to moderately better than standard nonsurgical therapy without intense rehab.
- In radiating pain from a herniated disc, there was good evidence that discectomy (surgery) was moderately better than nonsurgical treatment through 2-3 months after the operation. I think it's important to note that it is not clear, in fact it's doubtful, as to whether the researchers considered or compared conservative spinal decompression recovery and success rates to those of surgery.
- Let us keep that in mind before we accept that the surgery was "moderately better than nonsurgical treatment." In our experience here in my office, that would only be true in a handful of cases out of several hundred. They're just not looking at ALL of the information in this paper.
- They also found that benefits with surgery often decreased over the long-term when followed up on.

Wrap It Up

Surgery for radiating pain from a herniated disc and/or spinal stenosis that is actively hurting is associated with short-term benefits when compared to nonsurgical therapy. Although, as noted above, they aren't including ALL nonsurgical therapies when making this opinion. Most notably absent are safer and less invasive treatments like traction, mobilization, manipulation, etc.

For non-radiating back pain in the case of degeneration, fusion surgery is no more effective than intensive rehab[39].

LESS SURGERY WHEN GOING TO A CHIROPRACTOR FIRST

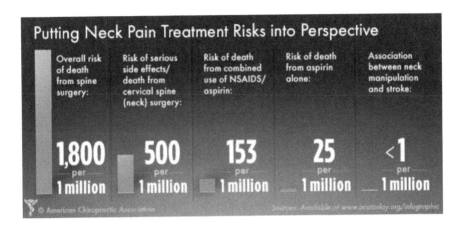

Putting Neck Pain Treatment Risks into Perspective

Overall risk of death from spine surgery:	Risk of serious side effects/ death from cervical spine (neck) surgery:	Risk of death from combined use of NSAIDS/ aspirin:	Risk of death from aspirin alone:	Association between neck manipulation and stroke:
1,800 per 1 million	**500** per 1 million	**153** per 1 million	**25** per 1 million	**<1** per 1 million

© American Chiropractic Association   Sources: Available at www.acatoday.org/infographic

Why Did They Do It?

To see if there were any predictors of whether a person would end up having low back surgery inside of 3 years after their work injury. Back injuries are the most common work injury and low back pain is the global leader in disability.

How Did They Do It?

- They used Disability Risk Identification Study Cohort (D-RISC) data
- They used baseline worker-reported measures from about 3 weeks after the injury claim was made.
- They used medical billing data to find out if they ever underwent the surgery inside of 3 years

- In the D-RISC sample of 1885 people, 174 of them had surgery within 3 years
- REDUCED ODDS OF SURGERY were noticed for people that were 35 years or younger, were female, were Hispanic, or whose FIRST PROVIDER WAS A CHIROPRACTOR.
- Around 42.7% of workers who saw a surgeon first had surgery. Only **1.5% of those seeing a chiropractor first had surgery[40].**

THE SECRET BEHIND LOW BACK SURGERY

Chiropractors see patients almost daily that are considering spinal surgery as a solution to their pain. Far too often, they perceive surgery as an early option rather than the **last** option. We are careful to advise our patients that there are only a few reasons to consider low back surgery initially.

There are certainly urgencies that require immediate surgical treatment. Things like myelopathy and atrophy require immediate attention. Progressive neurological deficits, caudal equina syndrome, and unrelenting, life-changing pain all need a serious second look and surgery certainly may be on the table for these patients.

In general, however, outside of conditions requiring immediate attention, surgery should always be the ultimate and final option.

This is not only because it is invasive and has serious risks of adverse events and a significant recovery period, but also because many surgeries must be repeated. Even in successful outcomes, the patient is likely to develop spinal conditions above and below the site of surgery as the years pass by.

In addition, when a patient suffers from chronic pain syndrome due to a hypersensitized central nervous system, they run a 60% chance of developing chronic pain at the new site of injury - even when the surgery goes perfectly.

Of course, there are lost causes and cases that are beyond helping conservatively, but we strongly believe there are better ways to go about treating spinal pain than surgery in general.

Why They Did It

Since low back pain is so common with medical appointments, and related surgeries remain controversial, as well as the fact that new techniques for surgery and treatment continue to emerge, the authors felt it important that low back pain treatment be evidence-based through solid research. They wanted to gather all the research they could find on low back surgery in order to analyze the outcomes, the quality of the research, and the conclusions of the research papers.

How They Did It

- The authors used available medical databases to search for research having to do with low back pain and surgical treatment.
- There were two different independent investigators.
- The quality of each research paper was assessed through professional, standardized questionnaires (AMSTAR and PRISMA).
- It was determined that none of the authors of this paper had any conflict of interest.
- The diagnoses in the paper were categorized separately as disc herniation, spondylolisthesis, stenosis, facet joint syndrome, and degenerative disc disease.

What They Found

- The authors included 40 reviews in this study.
- According to the quality questionnaires, only 5-7.5% of the papers were rated as excellent.
- Most of the research papers were rated as being of fair quality.

- In addition, 22.5% of the reviews (AMSTAR) were determined to be of very poor quality, while the other questionnaire (PRISMA) determined that 7.5% of the papers were of very poor quality.
- Ultimately, only 44% of the papers had a conclusion that was evidence-based, and 37.5% didn't even reach a conclusion on the primary objective.

Wrap It Up

Most systematic review papers on lower back pain and surgery don't reach very good or excellent quality. In fact, a mere 27.5% of them even contain evidence-based conclusions.

That simply does not bode well for those considering lower back surgery at this time[41].

RESEARCH: LUMBAR FUSION OUTCOMES

This study on low back fusion was done within the Washington State Workers' Compensation system.

Why They Did It

To find out how effective lumbar fusion surgery and devices were on clinical and disability outcomes. This was a question worth asking as the rates of lumbar fusions continue to increase.

How They Did It

- They identified injured workers from Washington State that had lumbar fusion between 1994 and 2001.
- They found these people through the Washington State Workers' Compensation system administrative database.
- They considered different factors such as specific technique, risk or disability, re-operation rates, and post-surgical complication.
- They found 1,950 people eligible for the study.

Jeff S. Williams, DC, FIANM

What They Found
- Of the 1,950 patients, fusions involving the installation of cages went up from 3.6% of the surgeries in 1996, to 58.1% of the surgeries in 2001.
- Overall disability rates at the 2-year (post-surgical) mark equaled 63.9%
- Re-operation rates for the same timetable were 22.1%
- Complications rate over the same period was 11.8%.
- Use of cages or instrumentation was associated with more risk of complication when compared to bone-only fusions.
- Discography and multilevel fusions predicted more re-operations.

Wrap It Up
New intervertebral fusion devices were introduced in 1996. These devices are associated with increased complications, re-operations, and disability[42].

ARE CHIROPRACTORS GREEDY & EXPENSIVE?

One of the misperceptions I hear from time to time is that chiropractors are greedy or that they just want to see how many times they can get a patient in and out of their doors based purely on financial gain.

Let's not beat around the bush here: there most certainly are opportunists in **EVERY** profession in the world. In my experience, chiropractic is no exception.

However, in general, people are good by nature and, again, chiropractors are no exception. Truly, the vast majority of chiropractors went into business to **help** people. No other reason. Just to help.

Before we dive into the research here, ask yourself a simple question, "If my primary family doctor sent me to a physical therapist, would they just see me once and then tell me to call if it keeps bothering me?"

If you've had any experience with physical therapy, you already know the answer to that question. Of course not! You'll be treated on a steady and consistent basis for a specific amount of time because any change in the body, or substantial healing, takes time and consistency.

In addition, building any significant durability to avoid future exacerbation or aggravation of the original injury or complaint is something that takes work. This is mostly common sense.

With that being said, let's dive in.

The Manga Report is an old chiropractic standard. This report has been around for some time now. Since 1993 to be exact.

Why They Did It
To assess the effectiveness in terms of physical recovery or pain alleviation as well as the cost-effectiveness of chiropractic in regards to treating low back pain.

How They Did It
The Ontario Ministry of Health-commissioned study was a comprehensive review of all of the published literature on low back pain.

What They Found
- They found an overwhelming amount of evidence showing the effectiveness of chiropractic in regard to the treatment of low back pain and complaint.
- They also found that chiropractic is more cost-effective than traditional medical treatment and management.
- Found that many of the traditional medical therapies used in low back pain are considered questionable and, although some are very safe, some can lead to other problems being suffered by the patient.

- There are no case-controlled studies that suggest chiropractic is not safe for the treatment of low back pain. They showed that chiropractic is clearly more cost-effective and that there would be highly significant savings if more low back pain management were controlled by chiropractors rather than medical physicians.
- The study stated that chiropractic services should be fully insured.
- The study stated that services should be fully integrated into the overall healthcare system due to the high cost of low back pain and the cost-effectiveness and physical effectiveness of chiropractic.
- They also stated that a good case could be made for making chiropractors the entry point into the healthcare system for musculoskeletal complaints that presented to hospitals.

Wrap It Up
Chiropractic should be the treatment of choice for low back pain, even excluding traditional medical care altogether[21]!

EXPERT PROOF FOR LOW BACK PAIN TREATMENT RECOMMENDATIONS

Why They Did It
The authors in this paper note that low back pain is 5th most common issue causing people to seek treatment at a doctor's office. They go on to state that about 25% of American adults experienced low back pain lasting an entire day at least one time in the previous three months. In addition, low back pain cost about $26.3 billion back in 1998.

The authors wanted to conduct a systematic review of the available evidence regarding the treatment of low back pain in adults.

How They Did It

- The data was collected via literature taken from sources such as MEDLINE, Cochrane Database of Systematic Reviews, the Cochrane Central Register of Controlled Trials, and EMBASE.
- The papers only contained randomized, controlled trials on patients having low back pain (with or without associated leg pain.
- The patients needed to have reported at least 1 of the following Outcome Assessments:
  back-specific function
  generic health status
  pain
  work disability
  patient satisfaction
- The American College of Physicians and the American Pain Society collaborated to create guidelines and procedure for the review and subsequent recommendations.

What They Found

- "For acute low back pain (duration <4 weeks), spinal manipulation administered by providers with appropriate training is associated with small to moderate short-term benefits.
- For chronic low back pain, moderately effective non-pharmacologic therapies include acupuncture, exercise therapy, massage therapy, Viniyoga-style yoga, cognitive-behavioral therapy or progressive relaxation, spinal manipulation, and intensive interdisciplinary rehabilitation."

Wrap It Up

Complementary and Alternative Medicine (CAM) protocols are absolutely effective for both long-term and acute low back pain and should be considered as an entry point into the healthcare system for mechanical low back pain[43].

HOW DO MEDICAL AND CHIROPRACTIC CARE STACK UP FOR LOW BACK PAIN?

Low back pain is one of the biggest issues seen in physical medicine and primary care clinics. There have been questions about the effectiveness of mechanical-assisted manipulation when compared to regular manual-thrust manipulation,,as well as to the effectiveness of manipulation compared to usual medical care.

Why They Did It
The authors in this study wanted to find out what the effectiveness was of the following treatment protocols:
1. Manual-thrust manipulation (MTM) vs. mechanical-assisted manipulation (MAM), and
2. Manual-thrust manipulation (MTM) vs. usual medical care (UMC)

How They Did It
- 107 adults with low back pain within 12 weeks
- Randomized the treatment groups into MTM, MAM, or UMC
- Measured outcomes with Oswestry Low Back Pain Questionnaire and the Numeric Pain Rating scale
- Patients in the manipulation groups were treated 2x/week for 4 weeks
- Patients in the UMC group were treated 3 times during the same time period.
- Outcome measurements were performed at the start, 4 weeks in, 3 months in, and then 6 months in.

What They Found
- There was a statistically significant advantage of Manual-Thrust Manipulation at 4 weeks compare with MAM and UMC.
- Similar results were found in regard to statistically significant pain reduction across the groups. Manual-thrust manipulation won the day.

Wrap It Up

Manual-Thrust Manipulation (a.k.a. – CHIROPRACTIC) shows statistically significant effectiveness short-term in self-reported outcome assessments when compared to usual medical care and mechanical assisted manipulation[44].

STUDIES RELATED TO THE LUMBAR (LOW BACK) REGION

DOES SPINAL MANIPULATION REALLY WORK ON LOW BACK PAIN?

"**B**ut my dad's old doctor told him that chiropractors don't work. He said that they'll just hurt you. He said Oooooh....you better be careful going to chiropractors."

Chiropractors around the nation hear comments like these almost weekly, and that is what makes this evidence-based effort necessary. People hold those old medical doctors in high regard, respect, and esteem. And, let's be honest, most of them have earned that respect over their lives of taking care of a community's needs for many years.

When you tell people that research suggests that medical doctor was speaking out of ignorance, they do not always believe what we are saying. Not only that, but some do not take too kindly to it (as they say in the South).

Fortunately, they do not have to believe me. But, they do need to believe the people that do the research. In many cases, it is medical doctors, PhDs, governments, universities, and insurance companies performing these research papers.

It is not just chiropractors getting together to tell people how good they are, to generate some meaningless research, and to pat each other on the back.

IN MANY CASES, IT IS THE LONG-TIME, TRADITIONAL ENEMIES OF CHIROPRACTORS THAT ARE TELLING YOU HOW GOOD ASPECTS OF CHIROPRACTIC CARE CAN BE!

Why Did They Do It?

As back pain is the leading cause of disability globally, the medical field know some answers need to be found. Four out of five adults experience and deal with back pain. The authors wanted to determine long-term outcomes of low back pain treatment.

They wanted to evaluate factors dealing with prognosis. They also wanted to contrast and compare medical treatment vs. chiropractic treatment in back and leg pain patients.

How Did They Do It?
1. 832 chiropractors
2. 111 medical doctors
3. Measured pain, disability, and satisfaction at 6 and at 12 months
4. They used the Visual Analog Scale and the Revised Oswestry Disability Questionnaire to determine progress or lack thereof.

What Did They Find?
- Long-term pain and disability were about the same in chiropractic and medical patients **BUT** there were significant differences. That's just the cover of the book. It's not the meat and potatoes.
- Chiropractic showed superior results when compared to traditional medical care for those with pain radiating below the knee associated with low back pain.
- Chiropractic patients were more satisfied with all parts of their care than were the medical patients.
- Wrap It Up
- Chiropractic wins in low back pain and pain radiating below the knee.
- Patients love their chiropractors more than they love their medical doctor[45].

AXIAL TRACTION FOR LOW BACK DISCS

"Effectiveness of Traction in Young Patients Representing Different Stages of Degenerative Disc Disease" authored by Kuligowski, et. al[46]and published in the Journal of Orthopedics, Traumatology, and Rehabilitation on June 30 of 2019.

Why They Did It

The authors say that traction techniques are a popular method of treating lumbar disc herniation. The type of lumbar disc herniation (protrusion, extrusion) in young people appears to determine patients' clinical status, necessitating diversification of treatment methods with regard to the type of damage.

How They Did It

- They enrolled 37 people aged 22-35
- The subjects had MRIs, which determined if they went to the protrusion group or the extrusion group
- During treatment, patients were in the supine position
- They were given three-dimensional traction using a manual therapy
- Oswestry questionnaire, MRC scale, Numeric Rating Scale, SLR test, Passive Lumbar Extension test and measurements of lumbar segment mobility were used for clinical evaluation.

What They Found

- An analgesic effect was noted with regard to the Oswestry and the Numeric Rating Scale. There were statistically significant differences observed in the case of parameters reflecting the subjective evaluation of disability and pain levels on the Outcome Assessments.
- These differences were clear and statistically significant with more pronounced changes observed in the group of patients with protrusions.

- The subjects improved clinically with regard to the Passive Lumbar Extension and the Straight Leg Raise.
- A statistically significant result was observed with regard to subjective pain levels on the NRS, again, with a better result in the protrusion group. Which I think is to be expected. Both groups improved in most measures with protrusion having the best results. But also keep in mind on the extrusions, outside of this paper, we know that an extrusion with migration is more likely to be self-absorbed by the body so it's not all doom and gloom even for the extrusion group.

Wrap It Up
1. The type of intervertebral disc damage determines the functional status of young people with degenerative disc disease.
2. The study demonstrated and confirmed a positive effect of traction on the functional status of subjects with lumbar disc herniation.
3. Traction techniques are safe and can be successfully used in the treatment of lumbar disc herniation.

ADJUSTMENTS – A REVIEW AND ANALYSIS OF THE AVAILABLE INFORMATION

First thing's first: this research discusses the adjustment using the term osteopathic manipulative treatment (OMT). This can be considered to be the same thing. There is no significant difference between the two.

In fact, for those in the audience that are strictly of the medical and osteopath mindset, it should, in your mind, legitimize the chiropractic adjustment since doctors of osteopathy learned spinal and joint manipulation in their respective schools as well.

Why Did They Do It?

They wanted to test spinal manipulation in low back pain to see how effective it is as a complementary treatment.

How Did They Do It?

1. They used searches of MEDLINE, EMBASE, MANTIS, OSTMED, and the Cochrane Central Register of Controlled Trials.
2. Identified six trials that had studies of eight blinded, controlled trials of OMT of low back disorder.
3. They used two independent reviewers to assess the information.
4. The trials included spinal manipulation vs. active treatment (i.e., traditional medical treatment) or placebo control.

What Did They Find?

- Spinal manipulation showed significant results in reducing low back pain.
- Significant reduction of pain occurred whether the study was performed in the United Kingdom or the United States.
- Significant pain reduction at **ALL** points of follow-up: short term, mid-term, and long-term

Wrap It Up

Spinal manipulation, **AGAIN**, is shown to be superior in reducing low back pain. It was even **MORE** effective than the researchers expected[47].

CHIROPRACTIC MANAGEMENT OF LOW BACK PAIN AND BACK-RELATED LEG PAIN

Why They Did It

To assess literature regarding the use of spinal manipulation in low back pain.

A search was done of available research from databases that included PubMed, Mantis, and the Cochrane Database. In addition, there was an invitation to healthcare professionals through association media to submit relevant articles for inclusion.

What They Found

887 source documents were found. These were filtered into categorized groups:
1. Randomized controlled trials (RCT)
2. Randomized trials of other interventions for low back pain
3. Guidelines
4. Systematic reviews
5. Basic Science
6. Diagnostic-related articles
7. Methodology
8. Cognitive therapy and psychosocial issues
9. Cohort and outcome studies

Wrap It Up

"As much or more evidence exists for the use of spinal manipulation to reduce symptoms and improve function in patients with chronic low back pain as for use in acute and sub-acute low back pain. Also, use of exercise in addition to manipulation will probably speed the case along and lead to even better outcomes while reducing instances of exacerbation of the condition[48].

DO YOU TRUST CONSUMER REPORTS?

As recently as 2011, Consumer Reports did a survey on 45,601 people. The survey was on alternative healthcare treatments and what technique/modality seemed the most helpful. They found that 3 out of 4 people were using some sort of alternative treatment to control their general health.

Manual therapies (hands-on) were the most utilized. Therapies such as chiropractic, massage, and yoga. They were widely used for conditions like back pain, arthritis, and neck pain.

In terms of back pain treatments, **Chiropractic outperformed all other forms of treatment, including prescription medication.**

It is very clear that, of the people that are actually utilizing Chiropractic, they are reporting that is has been significantly effective in treating their complaints! The following graphics are from the Consumer Reports website[49].

Back-pain treatments	% who used	% helped a lot
Chiropractic	36%	65%
Prescription medication	38	53
Deep-tissue massage	24	51
Yoga	9	49
Pilates	3	49
Acupressure	3	45
Swedish massage	6	41
Acupuncture	8	41
Shiatsu massage	3	36
Progressive relaxation	3	32
Meditation	5	29
Over-the-counter medication	58	28
Deep-breathing exercises	6	23
Magnesium supplements	4	15
Glucosamine/chondroitin	14	12
Vitamin D	8	10
Calcium supplements	10	9
Fish-oil supplements	10	7
Vitamin C	4	6
Multivitamins	11	5

Differences of less than 5 percentage points are not meaningful.

Neck treatments

Around six in 10 of those who used chiropractic or deep-tissue massage said it helped a lot as a neck treatment. But respondents rated Swedish massage and prescription medication a toss-up. Most people used over-the-counter medication, but only one in four said it helped a lot. And even fewer of those who used supplements thought they were beneficial.

What the research says

Some preliminary evidence suggests that spinal manipulation or a gentler version called mobilization, combined with exercise, can significantly reduce pain. Without exercise, the chiropractic treatments seem ineffective.

Precautions

Neck pain is usually gone within days or weeks. If it lasts longer or gets worse, see a doctor. Chiropractic procedures on the neck have been linked with severe side effects including stroke, which appears to be very rare.

Neck-pain treatments	% who used	% helped a lot
Chiropractic	41%	64%
Deep-tissue massage	35	58
Swedish massage	8	51
Prescription medication	33	49
Yoga	10	45
Acupuncture	10	44
Deep-breathing exercises	10	27
Over-the-counter medication	56	25
Glucosamine/chondroitin	13	14
Calcium supplements	11	6
Multivitamins	13	4

Differences of less than 7 percentage points are not meaningful.

Headache and migraine treatments

Readers rated prescription medications significantly more helpful than all other headache treatments. Most tried over-the-counter drugs, and just more than half said they helped a lot.

Headache treatments	% who used	% helped a lot
Prescription medication	43%	77%
Over-the-counter medication	78	51
Chiropractic	15	45
Deep-tissue massage	14	40
Acupuncture	6	34
Acupressure	4	32
Yoga	6	31
Meditation	9	21
Deep-breathing exercises	9	19
Progressive relaxation	5	18
Aromatherapy	4	18
Magnesium supplements	7	15

Differences of less than 3 percentage points are not meaningful.

Jeff S. Williams, DC, FIANM

COMPARISON OF COMBINED APPROACH TO ACUTE LOW BACK PAIN – 2011

This study was held in the UK in 2011 so the information is fairly recent. This study makes mention of a "stratified" primary care management protocol. This term is used to describe the use of alternative treatment (manual therapy).

As one reads through this paper, it would be appropriate to replace the word "stratified" with alternative treatments or manual therapy.

How They Did It

The authors were well aware that back pain remains a significant challenge for primary practitioners to treat and manage. They were also aware of the fact that co-management of back pain among primary practitioners and alternative therapies had yet to tested by them.

How They Did It.

- They compared effectiveness of treatment with the cost of the treatment between combined treatment and non-combined.
- They used 1573 adults over the age of 18 with either radiating symptoms or without.
- They were randomly placed into one of the two groups
- They used the Roland Morris Disability Questionnaire to assess the condition at the 12-month mark.

What Did They Find?

- Overall, the scores were "significantly higher in the intervention group than in the control group" at 4 months and at 12 months.
- At the 12 month mark, the combined care model showed an increase in "generic health benefit" AND "cost savings" when compared with the control group.

1. When properly screened and treated, a combined approach to treatment of acute low back pain "will have important implications for the future management of back pain in primary care[12]."

SHORT-TERM EFFECT OF CHIROPRACTIC SPINAL ADJUSTMENTS

Why They Did It
The reason for this research was to determine what the short-term effects of spinal manipulation are on males in regards to pain, spinal mobility or range of motion, and height recovery in the instance of degenerative disc disease following high-velocity, low-amplitude spinal manipulation in the low back/sacral region at L5/S1.

This research was performed in a University-based physical therapy, clinical setting and was a RANDOMIZED CONTROLLED DOUBLE BLIND trial performed by Vieira-Pellenz F, et al.

How They Did It:
The Gold Standard of research was applied here. It was randomized, controlled, and double blind starting with a baseline reading then measuring the results post-treatment.

There were forty male participants that had received the diagnosis of degenerative lumbar disc disease. This was a qualification for inclusion in the study.

There was a control group and a treating group. The treatment group received a single L5/S1 adjustment. The control group received "sham" treatment that the researchers knew would have no effect for the better or worse.

Measures:
- The patient's height was measured using a stadiometer.
- There was also a measurement of perceived low back discomfort with was measured via the visual analogue scale (VAS).
- The neural mechanosensitivity was measured via the Straight Leg Test (SLR).
- The amount of spinal mobility was measured in flexion using the finger to the floor distance test (FFD).

What They Found
There was a significant amount of improvement in all aspects of the Treatment Group while there were no changes at all in the Control Group except for a minimal improvement in the FFD (p=0.008).

Wrap It Up
Chiropractic spinal manipulation in the lower back region, when performed on males with degenerative disc disease, show immediate and significant improvement of perceived back pain (VAS), spinal mobility in flexion (FFD), hip flexion (SLR), and height (stadiometer) [50].

HOSPITAL-BASED STUDY SAYS CHIROPRACTIC MAY BE A BETTER ANSWER IN LOW BACK PAIN

Sometimes, as I'm making my way through the internet, certain articles that are not actually research papers, but based on research, will catch my eye. This article appeared in the Journal Dynamic Chiropractic.

It referred to research that came out in 2008 from Canada. It was discussing a program they put together in the hospitals in which patients were co-managed by medical doctors and chiropractors and it was written by Paul Bishop, MD, DC, PhD.

It was called the chiropractic hospital-based interventions research outcomes study. The argument was that there has been tons of research coming out in favor of chiropractors and spinal manipulative treatments but little has been accomplished toward implementing any new ideas or procedures in order to take advantage of the new knowledge gained from the research.

Basically, chiropractors still weren't getting referrals for cases even though research has shown time and time again that chiropractic is the treatment of choice. There remained a large gap between what medical providers THINK is effective and what actually IS effective according to research studies.

So, C.H.I.R.O. was set up as the "gold-standard, research-methodology clinical trials designed to evaluate the chiropractic assessment and treatment of patients with acute or chronic cervical, thoracic, or lumbosacral spine pain stratified by underlying spine pathology."

This was to be in a hospital-based setting at Orthopaedic and Neurosurgical Spine Program at Canada's National Spine Institute, in the Faculty of Medicine at the University of British Columbia in Vancouver.

The study was a randomized clinical trial and compared traditional medical care with "study care." The Study Care group included lumbar adjustments administered by chiropractors.

Wrap It Up
The patients experienced overall significantly better functional improvements and quality of life outcomes than traditional medical care alone[51].

ARE CHIROPRACTORS GREEDY & EXPENSIVE?

One of the misperceptions I hear from time to time is that chiropractors are greedy or that they just want to see how many times they can get a patient in and out of their doors based purely on financial gain.

Let's not beat around the bush here: there most certainly are opportunists in EVERY profession in the world. I'm certain that Chiropractic is no exception. So, every now and then, they may be right.

However people, in general, are good by nature and, again, chiropractors are no exception. Truly, the vast majority of chiropractors got into business to help people. No other reason. Just to help.

Before we dive into the research here, ask yourself a simple question, "If my primary sent me to a physical therapist, would they just see me once and then tell me to call if it keeps bothering me?" If you've had any experience with a physical therapist, you already know the answer to that question. Of course not! You'll be treated on a steady and consistent basis for a specific amount of time because any change in the body, or substantial healing, take time and consistency.

In addition, building any significant durability to avoid future worsening of the original injury or complaint is something that takes work. This is mostly common sense.

With that being said, let's dive in. The Manga Report is an old chiropractic stand-by. This report has been around for some time now.

It's been around since 1993 to be exact.

Why They Did It
To assess the effectiveness in terms of physical recovery or pain alleviation as well as the cost-effectiveness of chiropractic in regards to treating low back pain.

How They Did It

The Ontario Ministry of Health-commissioned study was a comprehensive review of all of the published literature on low back pain.

What They Found

It's astounding actually, ready for this?

- They found an overwhelming amount of evidence showing the effectiveness of chiropractic in regard to the treatment of low back pain and complaint.
- They also found that it is more cost-effective than traditional medical treatment and management.
- Found that many of the traditional medical therapies used in low back pain are considered questionable in validity and, although some are very safe, some can lead to other problems being suffered by the patient.
- There are no case controlled studies that even hint or suggest the chiropractic is not safe for the treatment of low back pain. They showed that chiropractic is clearly more cost-effective and that there would be highly significant savings if more low back pain management was controlled by chiropractors rather than medical physicians.
- The study stated that chiropractic services should be fully insured.
- The study stated that services should be fully integrated into the overall healthcare system due to the high cost of low back pain and the cost-effectiveness and physical effectiveness of chiropractic.
- They also stated that a good case could be made for making chiropractors the entry point into the healthcare system for musculoskeletal complaints that presented to hospitals.

Wrap It Up

Chiropractic should be the treatment of choice for low back pain, even excluding traditional medical care altogether[21]!

MANUAL THERAPY &
EXERCISE IN GENERAL LOW BACK PAIN

Why They Did It.

The researchers wanted to review all evidence they could find on different types of manual therapy used on different patients throughout different stages in non-specific, general low back pain. That sounds like a heck of a good reason to me.

How They Did It

The researchers used Medline, PEDro, Cochrane-Register-of-Controlled-Trials, and EMBASE for their data mining. The time span for the studies they used ran from January 2000 to April 2013. Thirteen years is a pretty solid sampling. The review of all of this literature was done while following the Cochrane and PRISMA guidelines so it was formatted accordingly.

1. 360 studies evaluated
1. Two stages of low back pain were used (acute-subacute and chronic)
1. Manual therapy types were subcategorized: MT1 (manipulation) and MT2 (soft tissue techniques and mobilization)
1. Also, there was a MT3 which was MT1 and MT2 combined
1. MT could be combined in usage with exercise or usual medical care.

What They Found

ACUTE-SUBACUTE LOW BACK PAIN

STRONG EVIDENCE – MT1 had strong evidence on its side compared to fake treatment. It was effective in the treatment of pain, function, and health improvement in the short-term (1-3 months).

MODERATE-STRONG EVIDENCE – MT1 and MT3 combined with usual medical treatment in comparison to usual medical treatment alone. MT1 and MT3 with medical treatment was MORE effective than medical treatment alone for pain, function, and over health in the short-term.

MODERATE EVIDENCE – MT3 with exercise or usual medical treatment compared to exercise and back-school. MT3 with exercise or usual medical treatment was superior for the quality-of-life in the short and long-term[52].

LESS SURGERY WHEN GOING TO A CHIROPRACTOR FIRST

Why Did They Do It?

To see if there were any predictors of whether a person would end up having low back surgery inside of 3 years after their work injury. Back injuries are the most common work injury.

How Did They Do It?
- They used Disability Risk Identification Study Cohort (D-RISC) data
- They used baseline worker-reported measures from about 3 weeks after the injury claim was made.
- They used medical billing data to find out if they ever underwent the surgery inside of 3 years
- What Did They Find Out?
- In the D-RISC sample of 1885 people, 174 of them had surgery within 3 years
- REDUCED ODDS OF SURGERY were noticed for people that were 35 years or younger, were female, were Hispanic, or whose FIRST PROVIDER WAS A CHIROPRACTOR.
- Around 42.7% of workers who saw a surgeon first has surgery.
- Only 1.5% of those seeing a chiropractor first had surgery[40].

HOW DOES MEDICAL CARE AND CHIROPRACTIC CARE STACK UP FOR LOW BACK PAIN?

Low back is one of the biggest issues that is treated in physical medicine and primary care clinics. There have been questions as to the effectiveness of Mechanical-Assisted Manipulation when compared to regular Manual-Thrust Manipulation as well as to the effectiveness of manipulation compared to Usual Medical Care.

Why They Did It
The authors in this study wanted to find out what the effectiveness was of the following treatment protocols:
- Manual-thrust manipulation (MTM) vs. mechanical-assisted manipulation (MAM), and
- Manual-thrust manipulation (MTM) vs. usual medical care (UMC)

How They Did It
- 107 adults with low back pain within 12 weeks
- Randomized the treatment groups into MTM, MAM, or UMC
- Measured outcomes with Oswestry Low Back Pain Questionnaire and the Numeric Pain Rating scale
- Patients in the manipulation groups were treated 2x/week for 4 weeks
- Patients in the UMC group were treated 3 times during the same time period.
- Outcome measurements were performed at the start, 4 weeks in, 3 months in, and then 6 months in.

What They Found
- There was a statistically significant advantage of Manual-Thrust Manipulation at 4 weeks compare with MAM and UMC.
- Similar results were found in regards to statistically significant pain reduction in across the groups. Manual-Thrust Manipulation won the day.

Manual-Thrust Manipulation (chiropractic) shows statistically significant effectiveness short-term relief in self-reported Outcome Assessments when compared to Usual Medical Care and Mechanical Assisted Manipulation[44].

SPINAL MANIPULATION CRUSHES DICLOFENAC IN LOW BACK PAIN DOUBLE BLINDED RANDOMIZED CONTROLLED TRIAL

Here is a double blinded randomized placebo-controlled trial.

Why They Did It

The authors were interested in effectiveness of spinal manipulation (in the chiropractic style) vs. the non-steroidal anti-inflammatory drug called Diclofenac vs. a simple placebo.

How They Did It

1. They had 101 patients with low back pain less the 48 hours old.
2. They used several very strict rules to include, or exclude, the patients.
3. The patients were randomized into three groups: a) Spinal manipulation and placebo/diclofenac b) Fake manipulation and diclofenac, c) fake manipulation and placebo-diclofenac.
4. Outcomes were registered by a second (and blinded) investigator to minimize bias.
5. The outcomes were self-reported and assessed physical disability, function, off-work time, and medication taken to alleviate symptoms.
6. The outcomes were taken 12 weeks afterward.

What They Found
- 37 Patients had chiropractic adjustments
- 38 received Diclofenac
- 25 had no active treatment
- The intervention groups were significantly superior to the control group

Wrap It Up
- The manipulation group was significantly better than the Diclofenac group.
- No adverse effects or harms were registered.

Spinal manipulation was clinically superior to placebo and significantly better than Diclofenac[53].

PREVENTING LOW BACK PAIN FROM RETURNING WITH A VENGEANCE

Some chiropractors simply are not able to employ physical rehabilitation as part of their practice. Many just do not have the space available to perform rehabilitation in a meaningful way. However, most will send exercises with the patient to be done on their own in the privacy of their homes. Our goal as patient-centered practitioners should be to enable patients to self-manage at home rather than depend solely on a practitioner of any sort.

Whether a chiropractor has patients actively performing rehabilitation or whether they encourage patients to be performing at-home exercises, exercise recommendations are a big part of common chiropractic treatment protocols.

Why They Did It
Not only is low back extremely common but, so is the recurrence of low back pain. The authors of this paper wanted to delineate

whether or not exercise intertwined into the treatment or as post-treatment was the most effective form of implementation and what was effective in preventing recurring low back pain.

How They Did It
- A comprehensive search was performed including CENTRAL (Cochrane Library 2009, Issue 3), MEDLINE, EMBASE, and CINAHL.
- The search was conducted up to the year 2009.
- Papers were accepted under specific criteria such as:
  - Subjects having had back pain before
  - An intervention that consisted of exercises alone
  - Outcomes measuring recurrence metrics
- Two authors independently reviewed the material for acceptance.
- The studies were divided into post-treatment intervention and treatment studies.
- Results were combined with meta-analyses of subjects, treatments, controls, and outcomes.

What They Found
- They ultimately reviewed 13 articles that reported on 9 studies with 9 interventions.
- Four studies had low risk of bias while one had a high risk. The others were undetermined.
- There was moderate evidence post-treatment exercise was more effective in reducing recurrence than was no treatment at the one year follow up.
- There was moderate evidence the recurrence rate was significantly reduced in two of the study at the 1.5 years and at the 2 years follow-ups.
- There was conflicting evidence as to whether or not exercise alone as a treatment protocol was effective.

Jeff S. Williams, DC, FIANM

Moderate quality evidence that post-treatment exercise programs can prevent recurrences of back pain but conflicting evidence found for exercise as the treatment itself.

Although this study was not intended to test the validity of physical therapy as a treatment itself, physical therapy is essentially exercise. The study suggests (to me) that physical therapy alone may not be the best protocol for low back pain and, in my opinion, could be better if combined with manual therapy and spinal mobilization[54].

WHY CHIROPRACTIC IS THE SECRET WEAPON FOR BACK & NECK PAIN

For some reason, regardless of the evidence and research out there in support of chiropractic, manual therapies, and spinal mobilization, there are those that continue to disparage the profession rather than educate themselves on its efficacy.

I believe that there are outliers in every industry, including our profession. Most people are sensible enough to understand that there are outlier plumbers that will take advantage of a person just because they're in the position to do so. There are mechanics changing perfectly good automotive parts and surgeons doing questionable or unnecessary surgery. There are insurance salesmen that will sell you insurance coverage they know will not really do you a lot of good. There are chiropractors out there that will make claims they should not make and will see you when it will not necessarily make much difference to your health.

I think it's understandable that outliers exist and avoiding them is just part of navigating through life. There's even a quote for it. "Fool me once, shame on you.....fool me twice, shame on me", right?

But it seems that outliers get more attention in the Chiropractic profession than do the highly educated and highly professional practitioners that are getting people well every single day. This is, for obvious reasons, highly frustrating.

It is only through continual and consistent sharing of the research and evidence that the Chiropractic profession will change and eventually overcome this situation. I have faith that solid research and evidence can only be ignored for a specific amount of time. There is a shelf-life, if you will, on its being ignored.

So, with that in mind, here's some research showing effectiveness of spinal manipulative therapy and/or mobilization for low back and neck pain.

Why They Did It
As said above, the authors felt that there were a multitude of randomized clinical trials, reviews, and national clinical guidelines regarding chiropractic for low back pain and neck pain but that there still remained some controversy as to the effectiveness among some in the medical field. They wanted to step back and review all of the information, only accept valuable papers on the topic, and generate a solid opinion on Chiropractic effectiveness for treating low back and neck pain.

How They Did It
1. They chose papers on randomized trials from around the world through computerized databases.
2. They used two independent reviewers to check the quality of the papers using guidelines laid out before starting the project.
3. 69 randomized clinical trials were reviewed.
4. Only 43 ultimately met the predetermined criteria and were accepted for the review.

- There is moderate evidence that Chiropractic has more effectiveness for short-term pain relief than does mobilization and limited evidence of faster recovery over physical therapy.
- For chronic low back pain, there is moderate evidence showing that spinal manipulative therapy has an effect that is equal to prescription nonsteroidal anti-inflammatory drug. Also, spinal manipulation and mobilization show effectiveness in short-term relief over that of a primary practitioner as well as superiority in the long term when compared to physical therapy.
- There is moderate to limited evidence showing that Chiropractic is superior to physical therapy in the long term and the short-term treatment of low back pain and neck pain.
- For a mix of short and long term pain, Chiropractic was either similar or superior to McKenzie exercises, medical treatment, or physical therapy.

Wrap It Up

The authors concluded that "recommendations can be made with confidence regarding the use of spinal manipulative therapy and/or mobilization as a viable option for the treatment of both low back pain and neck pain[33]."

WHAT WIKIPEDIA WON'T TELL YOU ABOUT CHIROPRACTIC

Patient Satisfaction. What exactly does that mean to you? Does that mean that you are feeling much better? Does that mean that you like the doctor? Does patient satisfaction mean that you were given very specific instructions and solid leadership about your treatment goals and protocols?

I think the answer is, "Yes." Yes to all of the above.

The research we're highlighting here does not necessarily have to do with whether a patient got better results from chiropractic when compared to some other form of treatment. There are plenty of other research papers proving that fact. However, it does speak to the fact that patients tend to be more satisfied with treatment and instruction given from a chiropractic physician.

Why They Did It
The authors wanted to attempt to understand differences in the level of patient satisfaction for patients that attended treatment with a chiropractor compared to those treated by a medical practitioner.

How They Did It
1. They measured standard satisfaction scores at the 4-week post-treatment point.
2. They used 672 randomized patients.

What They Found

The satisfaction scores for patients treated by the chiropractor were greater.

Wrap It Up
They said, "Communication of advice and information to patients with low back pain increases their satisfaction with providers and accounts for much of the difference between chiropractic and medical patients' satisfaction[55]."

LOW BACK DISCS: SURGICAL OR CONSERVATIVE CARE?

According to a paper by Donald Murphy, DC (And brought to my attention by Craig Benton, DC in Lampasas, TX), the following stats are scary but true:

- Between 1997 and 2005 – spending on spine-related disorders rose 65%.
- Between 1994-2004 – Medicare costs rose 629% for epidural steroid injections.
- Opioid medications rose 423%
- Spine MRIs rose 307%
- Lumbar fusion surgeries rose 220%

At the same time, there have been fewer positive results or outcomes for people. Through outcome assessment tracking, and self-reports, patients have shown a rise in physical limitations from 20.7% in 1997 to 24.7% in 2005. The number of disabled workers rose as well.

That's an amazing amount of additional expense and treatment, while providing less benefit. That is usually the point when a consumer starts to shop for alternatives in any other marketplace outside of the healthcare industry.

It is my opinion that conservative care should be tried first while taking a team approach amongst different practitioners as the best course of treatment. Now, on to the paper.

Why They Did It
See discussion above!

What Did They Decide?

Patients should first be screened for red flags and signs of surgical intervention such as:

- Bowel or bladder symptoms
- Fever
- Cancer
- Strange weight loss, etc...

<u>Absent of significant red flags, conservative treatment should be the entry point into the healthcare system.</u>

Wrap It Up

In addition to deciding that conservative treatment was the best initial option, of the conservative treatments available, chiropractic "has been shown through multiple studies to be safe, clinically effective, cost-effective, and to provide a high degree of patient satisfaction.

As a result, in patients with discogenic or radicular pain syndromes for whom the surgical indications are not absolute, a minimum of 2 or 3 months of chiropractic management is indicated[56]."

CHIROPRACTIC ADJUSTMENTS FOR LUMBAR DISC HERNIATIONS?

This isn't research performed in an attempt to say that chiropractic adjustments can "cure" a lumbar disc herniation. That is not what is being advocated in this entry.

In 2014, research showed that chiropractic adjustments were equal in effectiveness and patient outcome assessments as epidural steroid injections.

A separate paper also showed in 2014 that epidural steroid injections were strictly for short-term relief of inflammation caused by a herniated disc but had no effect on the disc itself. The paper also stated that there was absolutely no long-term effect from the injections on disability or as to whether or not a patient ended up having surgery.

Keeping these research papers in mind, one would have to advocate the use of chiropractic manipulation/mobilization with the goal of reducing inflammation caused by a lumbar herniation and increasing the mobilization of the segment to promote better blood flow, proprioception, and pain inhibition.

One would also reasonably estimate that chiropractic adjustments alone are unlikely to completely "cure" a herniated lumbar disc. It is for this reason that, for some doctors of chiropractic, the main course of treatment for lumbar disc herniation is non-surgical spinal decompression.

Why They Did It
They performed the study to estimate the effectiveness of chiropractic adjustments in patients that had lumbar disc herniations that were confirmed through the use of MRI imaging. They wanted to see if there was a difference between those conditions that were acute and chronic.

How They Did It
- It was a prospective cohort study.
- 148 patients included.
- Patients were between 18 and 65
- All had low back pain
- All had leg pain
- All had lumbar herniations that were confirmed through MRI imaging
- Outcomes were through self-assessed questionnaires at different time periods

- There was significant improvement on all outcome assessment questionnaires for all time intervals.
- 3 months post-treatment, 90.5% of patients were "improved"
- 1 year post-treatment, 88% were "improved"
- "Although acute patients improved faster by 3 months, 81.8% of chronic patients reported "improvement" with 89.2% "improved" at 1 year. There were no adverse events reported."

Wrap It Up

"A large percentage of acute and importantly chronic lumbar disc herniation patients treated with chiropractic spinal manipulation reported clinically relevant improvement[57]."

EVER HAD A CHIROPRACTOR TELL YOU TO COME BACK?

Why They Did It

The authors were curious as to whether there was any real, measured benefit to continued "maintenance" or "wellness" visits **beyond the initial phase of care** in regards to CHRONIC low back pain.

It's a great question that needed to be asked because patients come into our offices concerned about having to come see a chiropractor a million times, etc.

One of the old myths about chiropractic that can be heard periodically is that once you go to a chiropractor, you always have to go to a chiropractor. This simply is not true

However, it is reasonable to expect some consistency in treatment in the early going of a case. As with anything having to do with the musculoskeletal system, time and consistency are typically part of the process.

How They Did It
1. Single blinded, placebo-controlled
2. 60 patients
3. All chronic
4. They had to have suffered from the pain for at least 6 months.
5. Randomized to receive either
   - 12 adjustments of fake treatment over a 1-month period or
   - 12 treatments of actual treatments over a 1-month period with no treatment in the following nine months.
   - 12 treatments of actual treatments over a 1-month period followed by manipulation every 2 weeks for the next 9 months.

They measured pain and disability scores, generic health status, and back-specific patient satisfaction at 1 month, 4 month, 7 month, and 10-month intervals.

What They Found
Patients in the manipulation groups had significantly less pain and disability than did the first group when the 1 month period was up.

Only the third group (the one with follow up maintenance treatment) showed more improvement in these scores at the 10-month evaluation.

Wrap It Up
This study indicates that maintenance spinal manipulation offers the best long-term benefit[11].

Jeff S. Williams, DC, FIANM

SACROILIAC DYSFUNCTION

WHAT TREATMENT WORKS FOR PELVIC-RELATED LEG PAIN?

Why They Did It

The authors felt that sacroiliac joints (SIJ) could potentially be a source of sciatica. The goal of the study was to test whether there was a successful treatment regimen for a complaint of this sort.

How They Did It
- 51 patients with SIJ related leg pain were accepted into the study
- The study was a single-blinded randomized trial.
- Three treatment protocols were assessed in this study:
  - Physical Therapy/Physiotherapy
  - Chiropractic/Manual Therapy
  - Intra-articular corticosteroid injections
- The subjects were evaluated for improvement at the 6-week mark and at the 12-week mark.

What They Found
- Physical Therapy/Physiotherapy had a 20% success rate.
- Intra-articular corticosteroid injections had a 50% success rate.
- Chiropractic/Manual Therapy had a **72% success rate.**

Wrap It Up

"...manual therapy appeared to be the choice of treatment for patients with SIJ-related leg pain. A second choice of treatment to be considered is an intra-articular injection[58]."

I would like to add that the vast majority of chiropractors utilize exercise/rehabilitation as a significant part of their treatment protocols. Knowing this, it would be appropriate to point out the fact that chiropractors had a 72% success rate in this study while physical therapists had a 20% success rate. One would wonder what the success rate is when chiropractors COMBINE their treatment with physical therapy.

THE MOST EFFECTIVE MEANS OF TREATING SACROILIAC PAIN

Why They Did It

This study was all about chiropractic manipulation. Specifically, the authors wanted to know which was more effective for sacroiliac joint syndrome. Was the more effective treatment lumbar manipulation or sacroiliac joint manipulation (SIJ)?

How They Did It
- The study included 32 women diagnosed with SIJ dysfunction.
- The subjects were randomized evenly into 2 different groups.
- The treatment protocol for one group consisted of chiropractic adjustment to the involved SI joint.
- The second group's treatment protocol consisted of chiropractic adjustment and lumbar (low back) chiropractic adjustment in the same appointment.
- Outcome Assessment measurements were made through the use of the visual analogue scale (VAS) and the Oswestry Disability Index (ODI) questionnaire.
- The Outcome Assessment measurements were taken at the baseline mark, 48 hours post-treatment, and at the one-month post-treatment points.

What They Found

- The SI manipulation alone group showed statistically significant improvement at all points of Outcome Assessment measurement.
- Likewise, the SI manipulation AND Lumbar manipulation group showed a significant improvement at all points of Outcome Assessment measurement.

Wrap It Up

"A single session of SIJ and lumbar manipulation was more effective for improving functional disability than SIJ manipulation alone in patients with SIJ syndrome. Spinal HVLA manipulation may be a beneficial addition to treatment for patients with SIJ syndrome[59]."

Jeff S. Williams, DC, FIANM

STUDIES RELATED TO THE CERVICAL (NECK) REGION

TMJ THE RIGHT WAY

"Effect of Manual Therapy and Therapeutic Exercise Applied to the Cervical Region on Pain and Pressure Pain Sensitivity in Patients with Temporomandibular Disorders: A Systematic Review and Meta-analysis" authored by La Touche, et. al[60]. and published in Pain Medicine on March 17 of 2020.

Why They Did It
To assess the effectiveness of cervical manual therapy (MT) on patients with temporomandibular disorders (TMDs) and to compare cervico-craniomandibular manual therapy vs cervical manual therapy.

How They Did It
- The first thing that jumps out at me on this paper is that it is a systematic review and meta-analysis which means it's at the top of the research pyramid so it can be considered good information.
- They searched PubMed, EMBASE, PEDro, and Google Scholar with and end date of February 2019
- Two independent reviewers performed the data analysis and assessed the relevance of the randomized clinical trials

What They Found
- For cervical manual therapy, they included three studies that showed statistically significant differences in pain intensity reduction and an increase in master pressure pain thresholds, with a large clinical effect

- Also the results showed an increase in temporalis pressure pain thresholds with a moderate clinical effect
- The Meta-analysis included two studies on cervical manual therapy vs. cervico-craniomandibular manual therapy and showed statistically significant differences in pain intensity reduction and pain-free maximal mouth opening, with large clinical effect.

Wrap It Up

The authors wrapped their thoughts up by concluding "Cervical manual therapy treatment is more effective in decreasing pain intensity than placebo manual therapy or minimal intervention, with moderate evidence. Cervico-craniomandibular interventions achieved greater short-term reductions in pain intensity and increased pain-free motion over cervical intervention alone in TMJ/TMD and headache. Low evidence."

MANUAL THERAPY EFFECTIVENESS.

Does it REALLY Help?

This research is fairly recent being from 2010. It gives a good, general idea of the effectiveness of manual therapies. I would say it is one of the most important of the research abstracts to come out.

Why They Did It

The authors on this paper wanted to round up all the information they could find and bring it to one place for the purpose of evaluating how effective manual therapies are for lots of different musculoskeletal and non-musculoskeletal complaints. Basically, they wanted a comprehensive report on the chiropractic "goods."

How They Did It
- There was a full review of randomized clinical trials
- The strength and quality of the outcomes (effectiveness) was rated on a grading system.

What They Found
"Spinal manipulation/mobilization is effective in adults for: acute, subacute, and chronic low back pain; migraine and cervicogenic headache; cervicogenic dizziness; manipulation/mobilization is effective for several extremity joint conditions; and thoracic manipulation/mobilization is effective for acute/subacute neck pain." Also, "Massage is effective in adults for chronic low back pain and chronic neck pain."

Wrap It Up
Chiropractic is effective in acute, subacute, and chronic low back pain, migraines and headaches originating from the neck, for the treatment of some forms of dizziness, extremity and joint issues, as well as mid back and acute and subacute neck pain[61].

MANUAL THERAPY MORE EFFECTIVE, LESS EXPENSIVE

This research goes a **LONG WAY** towards showing the **cost-effectiveness** and the **overall effectiveness** of manual therapy/spinal mobilization when compared to traditional medical treatment or physiotherapy/physical therapy alone.

There is research out there that also shows extreme effectiveness through a combined, integrated approach in many musculoskeletal conditions.

Why They Did It

The authors wanted to evaluate, contrast, and compare effectiveness of manual therapy to physiotherapy/physical therapy and to care by a general medical practitioner in regards to neck pain specifically.

How They Did It

- This was an economic evaluation in addition to a randomized controlled trial.
- 183 Participants with neck pain for 2 weeks in duration
- 42 General medical practitioners
- The patients were randomly treated with manual therapy/ spinal mobilization, physiotherapy/physical therapy, or general practitioner protocols
- Clinical results were based on perceived recovery, intensity of pain, functional disability, and quality of life changes.
- Cost-efficiency was determined by the patients' keeping a log of costs for one year.

What They Found

Manual therapy/spinal mobilization shown to be faster in regards to improvement than BOTH physiotherapy/physical therapy and general practitioner protocols for up to 26 weeks.

The cost of manual therapy/spinal mobilization therapy were roughly 1/3 the cost of physiotherapy/physical therapy and general practitioner protocols.

Wrap It Up

Manual therapy/spinal mobilization was proven through research to be significantly more effective and cost less in the treatment of neck pain when compared to physiotherapy/physical therapy and general practitioners[27].

CHIROPRACTIC PROVEN EFFECTIVE FOR CERVICAL PAIN (SHORT AND LONG-TERM)

WHY THEY DID IT

The goal of the paper is to generate a comprehensive understanding about the effectiveness of manual therapy for musculoskeletal and non-musculoskeletal complaints.

HOW THEY DID IT
- Based on systematic reviews of only RANDOMIZED clinical trials. (The research Gold Standard basically)
- The trials had to be widely accepted and primarily UK and USA based guidelines used.

WHAT THE FOUND
- Spinal manipulation/mobilization is effective in adults for the following:
- Acute, subacute, and chronic low back pain
- Migraines
- Cervicogenic headaches
- Cervicogenic dizziness
- Several extremity joint conditions
- Acute or subacute neck pain

Wrap It Up

"Spinal manipulation/mobilization is effective in adults for: acute, subacute, and chronic low back pain; migraine and cervicogenic headache; cervicogenic dizziness; manipulation/mobilization is effective for several extremity joint conditions; and thoracic manipulation/mobilization is effective for acute/subacute neck pain. The evidence is inconclusive for cervical manipulation/mobilization alone for neck pain of any duration, and for manipulation/mobilization for mid back pain, sciatica, tension-type headache, coccydynia, temporomandibular joint disorders, fibromyalgia, premenstrual syndrome, and pneumonia in older adults. Spinal manipulation is not effective for asthma and dysmenorrhea when compared to sham manipulation, or for Stage 1 hypertension when added to an antihypertensive diet. In children, the evidence is inconclusive regarding the effectiveness for otitis media and enuresis, and it is not effective for infantile colic and asthma when compared to sham manipulation."[61].

A COUPLE OF WAYS TO DECREASE YOUR NECK PAIN

Here's a study from 2011 about neck pain treatment. It's a randomized controlled study showing the effectiveness of cervical manipulation and cold laser (low level laser) treatment for facet dysfunction.

Why They Did It
The goal was to find out the effectiveness of cervical manipulation combined with cold laser for the treatment of cervical facet syndrome. This condition is a common trigger for neck pain in otherwise healthy individuals.

How They Did It
- 6 women were accepted into the study.
- Their ages ranged between 18 and 40 yrs old.
- They all suffered from cervical facet joint pain lasting more than 30 days.
- Their treatments were randomized into 3 different protocol groups:
  ◦ Manipulation (Chiropractic)
  ◦ Cold laser
  ◦ A combination of the two treatments
- The following Outcome Assessments were used to measure the results and effectiveness:

- ◦ Numeric Pain Rating Scale
- ◦ Neck Disability Index
- ◦ Cervical Range of Motion Instrument
- ◦ Baseline Digital Inclinometer
- Measurements were taken in weeks 1, 2, 3, and 4.

What They Found
Significant improvements were found among all treatment groups, but the improvements were most noticeable in group three.

Wrap It Up
All three groups showed improvement, but a combination of manipulation and cold laser proved most effective. Both are proven to be viable treatment protocols for cervical facet syndrome[62].

CHIROPRACTIC MORE COST-EFFECTIVE AND MORE EFFECTIVE OVERALL THAN GENERAL PRACTITIONER

Why They Did It
The authors of this paper aimed to perform a review of trial-based economic evaluations that have been performed for manual therapy in comparison to other treatment protocols used for treatment of musculoskeletal complaints.

How They Did It
- The authors performed a comprehensive literature search of commonly used research databases for all subjects relative to this subject.
- 25 publications were included.
- The studies included cost-effectiveness for manual therapies compared to other forms of treatment for pain.
- What They Found
- Manual therapy techniques such as chiropractic mobilization were more cost effective than visiting a general practitioner.

- Specifically, chiropractic treatment was less costly and was found to be more effective than physiotherapy/physical therapy and visiting a General Practitioner's medical office when treating neck pain.

Wrap It Up

Although improvement in our knowledge of manual therapies is warranted, this paper demonstrates that Chiropractic is more cost-effective and more effective in general for low back pain & shoulder disability than usual medical practitioner care and physical therapy/physiotherapy[25].

CHRONIC NECK PAIN & REHAB EXERCISES

We see a good amount of research regarding the positive effects of spinal manipulation for low back pain. More specifically, we often see research for acute and chronic low back pain. This paper, however, spotlights the benefits of spinal manipulation in chronic neck pain. It covers not only the benefits of spinal manipulation, but also the addition of rehab exercises as part of the treatment regimen.

Why They Did It

The authors wanted to contrast the effectiveness of spinal manipulation when combined with low-tech rehab, MedX rehab, or spinal manipulation alone over the course of 2 years. Of the research available, the authors did not feel that there was adequate research outside of short-term follow-ups.

How They Did It
- 191 patients with chronic neck pain
- Patients were randomized to 11 weeks in one of the three treatment protocols.
- The patients self-reported on questionnaires measuring pain, disability, general health status, improvement, satisfaction, and medication use.

- The questionnaires were collected after 5 and 11 weeks of treatment
- They were also collected after 3, 6, 12, and 24 months after treatment concluded

What They Found
- 93% of the patients finished the 11 weeks of treatment.
- 76% provided the required information at all points of treatment and follow-up.
- There was a difference in the patient-rated pain in favor of the two exercise groups
- There was a difference in satisfaction with care when spinal manipulation was combined with rehab exercises.

Wrap It Up
There was a clear advantage of spinal manipulation combined with exercise vs. spinal manipulation alone over two years. The researchers concluded that chronic neck pain patients should enter treatment protocols including rehab exercises along with spinal manipulation for optimal results[63].

WHY CHIROPRACTIC IS THE SECRET WEAPON FOR BACK & NECK PAIN

Why They Did It
As said above, the authors felt that there were a multitude of randomized clinical trials, reviews, and national clinical guidelines regarding chiropractic for low back pain and neck pain but that there still remained some controversy as to the effectiveness among some in the medical field. They wanted to step back and review all of the information, only accept valuable papers on the topic, and generate a solid opinion on chiropractic effectiveness for treating low back and neck pain.

How They Did It
- They chose papers on randomized trials from around the world through computerized databases.
- They used two independent reviewers to check the quality of the papers using guidelines laid out before starting the project.
- 69 randomized clinical trials were reviewed.
- Only 43 ultimately met the predetermined criteria and were accepted for the review.

What They Found
- There is moderate evidence that Chiropractic has more effectiveness for short-term pain relief than does mobilization and limited evidence of faster recovery over physical therapy.
- For chronic low back pain, there is moderate evidence showing that spinal manipulative therapy has an effect equal to prescription non-steroidal anti-inflammatory drug. Also, spinal manipulation and mobilization show effectiveness in short-term relief over that of a primary practitioner as well as superiority in the long term when compared to physical therapy.
- There is moderate to limited evidence showing that Chiropractic is superior to physical therapy in the long term and the short-term treatment of low back pain and neck pain.
- For a mix of short and long term pain, Chiropractic was either similar or superior to McKenzie exercises, medical treatment, or physical therapy.

Wrap It Up
The authors concluded that "recommendations can be made with confidence regarding the use of spinal manipulative therapy and/or mobilization as a viable option for the treatment of both low back pain and neck pain[33]."

STUDIES RELATED
TO STROKE RISK

CERVICAL MANIPULATION.
WHAT YOU NEED TO KNOW

I have spent some serious time going through research, compiling lists, and battling with certain factions of the medical field that is strictly against any treatment involving cervical chiropractic adjustments. The common thread this group seems to always come back to is an imaginary notion that cervical manipulation is dangerous and is being performed for very little pay-off in the form of pain relief or reduction of disability.

This is simply untrue.
As I've stated many times, the relationship between the chiropractic and the medical fields has improved immensely, so please understand that I am referring to an antiquated part of the medical field that has remained stubborn and ignorant to current research. Some people just don't take to change of any sort.

However, if some in the medical field hold this idea, then there may be many in the public sector that have never been properly updated on how good (or bad) chiropractic can be for cervical musculoskeletal complaints.

It's in this spirit that I have compiled the following information. It includes studies that have accurately proven the benefits for cervical musculoskeletal complaints, headaches, migraines, and range of motion while also showing some of the research dispelling all claims of any real risk of stroke as a result.

All of these citations can be searched at PubMed online and read for further clarification if one strikes your interest. Also, at the very end of this section, I have included an article from the British Medical Journal just to put the period on the sentence.

I truly hope the following information can dispel some of the misinformation floating around and helps you in your decision to adopt Chiropractic as part of your regular healthcare regimen.

The most recent paper on the topic is by Chaibi, et. al.[64] It is titled "A risk-benefit assessment strategy to exclude cervical artery dissection in spinal manual-therapy: a comprehensive review", is authored by Aleksander Chaibi and Michael Bjorn Russell, and published in the March 2019 edition of the Journal of the Annals of Medicine.

Conclusion: "....... the reality is (a) that there is no firm scientific basis for direct causality between cervical SMT and CAD; (b) that the ICA moves freely within the cervical pathway, while 74% of cervical SMTs are conducted in the lower cervical spine where the VA also moves freely; (c) that active daily life consists of multiple cervical movements including rotations that do not trigger CAD, as is true for a range of physical activities; and (d) that a cervical manipulation and/or grade C cervical mobilization goes beyond the physiological limit but remains within the anatomical range, which theoretically means that the artery should not exceed failure strain. These factors underscore the fact that no serious AE was reported in a large prospective national survey conducted in the UK that assessed all AEs in 28,807 chiropractic treatment consultations, which included 50,276 cervical spine manipulations."

Research citations demonstrating efficacy of cervical manipulation/ mobilization in cervical pain and/or headache/migraine with citations demonstrating little to no risk of vertebral basilar artery dissection.

Cervical Studies

- Korthals-de Bos IB, et al. Cost effectiveness of physiotherapy, manual therapy, and general practitioner care for neck pain: economic evaluation alongside a randomised controlled trial. Randomized controlled trial British Medical Journal. 2003 Apr 26;326(7395):911.
- Dewitte V, Beernaert A, Vanthillo B, Barbe T, Danneels L, Cagnie B. Articular dysfunction patterns in patients with mechanical neck pain: A clinical algorithm to guide specific mobilization and manipulation techniques. Man Ther. 2014; 19(1):2-9.
- Dunning JR, Cleland J, Waldrop M, Arnot C, Young I, Turner M, Sigurdsson G. Upper cervical and upper thoracic thrust manipulation versus nonthrust mobilization in patients with mechanical neck pain: a multicenter randomized clinical trial. J Orthop Sports Phys Ther. 2012; 42(1): 5-18.
- Bronfort G, Evans R, AndersonA, Svendsen K, Bracha Y, Grimm R. Spinal Manipulation, Medication, or Home Exercise With Advice for Acute and Subacute Neck Pain: A Randomized Trial. Annals of Internal Medicine. 2012; 156(1): 1-10.
- Puentedura EJ, Cleland JA, Landers MR, Mintken PE, Louw A, Fernández-de-Las-Peñas C. Development of a clinical prediction rule to identify patients with neck pain likely to benefit from thrust joint manipulation to the cervical spine. J Orthop Sports Phys Ther. 2012; 42(7):577–92.
- Martínez-Segura R, De-la-Llave-Rincón AI, Ortega-Santiago R, Cleland JA, Fernández-de-Las-Peñas C. Immediate changes in widespread pressure pain sensitivity, neck pain, and cervical range of motion after cervical or thoracic thrust manipulation in patients with bilateral chronic mechanical neck pain: a randomized clinical trial. J Orthop Sports Phys Ther. 2012; Sep; 42(9):806–14.
- Yu H, Hou S, Wu W, He X. Upper cervical manipulation combined with mobilization for the treatment of atlantoaxial osteoarthritis: a report of 10 cases. J Manipulative Physiol Ther. 2011; 34(2):131-7.

- Puentedura EJ, Landers MR, Cleland JA, Mintken PE, Huijbregts P, Fernandez-de-Las-Penas C. Thoracic spine thrust manipulation versus cervical spine thrust manipulation in patients with acute neck pain: a randomized clinical trial. J Orthop Sports Phys Ther. 2011 ed. 2011; Apr;41(4):208–20.
- Leaver AM, Maher C, Herbet R, Latimer J, MacAuley J, Jull G. Refshauge K. A randomized controlled trial comparing manipulation with mobilization for recent onset neck pain. Arch Phys Med Rehabil. 2010; 91(9): 1313-8.
- Cleland, JA, Mintken PE, Carpenter K, Fritz JM, Glynn P, Whitman J, Childs JD. Examination of a clinical prediction rule to identify patients with neck pain likely to benefit from thoracic spine thrust manipulation and a general cervical range of motion exercise: Multi-center randomized clinical trial. Physical Therapy, 2010; 90(9): 1239-1250.
- Miller J, Gross A, D'Sylva J, Burnid SJ, Goldsmith CH, Graham N, Haines T, Gronfort G, Hoving JL. Manual therapy and exercise for neck pain: A systematic review. Manual Therapy, 2010; 15: 334-354.
- Gonzalez-Iglesia J, Fernandez-de-las-Penas C, Cleland JA, Alburquerque-Sendin F, Palmerque-del-Cerro F, Mendez-Sanchez R. Inclusion of thoracic spine thrust manipulation into an electrotherapy/thermal program for the management of patients with acute mechanical neck pain: a randomized trial. Manual Therapy, 2009; 14, 306-313.
- Hurwitz EL, Carragee EJ, van der Welde G, Carrol LJ, Nordin M, Guzman J, et al. Treatment of neck pain: noninvasive interventions: results of the Bone and Joint decade 2000-2010 task force on neck pain and its associated disorders. Spine 2008; 33(4 supplement) S123-S152.
- Fernandez-de-las-Penas C, Palomeqque-del-Cerro OL, Rodriguew-Blanco C, Comex-Conesa A, Miangolarra-Page JC. Changes in neck pain and active range of motion after a single thoracic spine manipulation in subjects presenting with mechanical neck pain: a case series. JMPT, 2007; 30(4): 312-320.
- Reinhold Muller and Lynton GF. "long-term follow-up of a randomized clinical trial assessing the efficacy of

medication, acupuncture, and spinal manipulation for chronic mechanical spinal pain syndromes. Journal of Manipulative and Physiological Therapeutics. 2005;28:3-11

- Zhu L, et al. "Does cervical spine manipulation reduce pain in people with degenerative cervical radiculopathy? A systematic review of the evidence, and a meta-analysis." Clin Rehabil. 2015 Feb 13.

- Giles LG, Muller R, "Chronic spinal pain a randomized clinical trial comparing medication, acupuncture, and spinal manipulation." Spine. 2003;28(14)/1490-1502

- Bronfort G, et al, "Efficacy of spinal manipulation and mobilization for low back pain and neck pain: a systematic review and best evidence synthesis." Spine. 2004;335-356.

- Hurwitz E, et al. "A randomized trial of chiropractic manipulation and mobilization for patients with neck pain: clinical outcomes from the UCLA neck pain study." Am Journal of Public Health. 2002;92:1634-1641.

- Saayman L, Hay C, Abrahamse H. "Chiropractic manipulative therapy and low-level laser therapy in the management of cervical facet dysfunction: a randomized controlled study. Randomized controlled trial" J Manipulative Physiol Ther. 2011 Mar-Apr;34(3):153-63.

- Snodgrass SJ, Rivett DA, Sterling M, Vicenzino B. "Dose optimization for spinal treatment effectiveness: a randomized controlled trial investigating the effects of high and low mobilization forces in patients with neck pain. Randomized controlled trial" J Orthop Sports Phys Ther. 2014 Mar;44(3):141-52.

- Buzzatti L, et al. "Atlanto-axial facet displacement during rotational high-velocity low-amplitude thrust: An in vitro 3D kinematic analysis." Man Ther. 2015.

Headache/Migraine Efficacy

- Nelson CF, Bronfort G, Evans R, et al. The efficacy of spinal manipulation, amitriptyline and the combination of both therapies for prophylaxis of migraine headache. Journal of Manipulative and Physiological Therapeutics, Oct. 1998;21(8), pp511-19. [36]

- Tuchin PJ, Pollard H, Bonello R. A randomized controlled trial of chiropractic spinal manipulative therapy for migraine. Journal of Manipulative and Physiological Therapeutics, Feb. 2000:23(2), pp91-5.
- Brontfort G, et. al. "Efficacy of spinal manipulation for chronic headache: a systematic review." J Manipulative Physiol Ther. 2001 Sep;24(7):457-66.
- Duke University Evidence-based Practice Center. Behavioral and physical treatments for tension-type and cervicogenic headache. Des Moines, IA: Foundation for Chiropractic Education and Research;2001.

Stroke Risk

- Kosloff TM, et al. "Chiropractic care and the risk of vertebrobasilar stroke: results of a case-control study in U.S. commercial and Medicare Advantage populations. Chiropr Man Therap. 2015 Jun 16;23:19.
- Whedon JM, et al. "Risk of stroke after chiropractic spinal manipulation in medicare B beneficiaries aged 66 to 99 years with neck pain." J Manipulative Physiol Ther. 2015 Feb;38(2):93-101.
- Achalandabaso A, et al. "Tissue damage markers after a spinal manipulation in healthy subjects: a preliminary report of a randomized controlled trial." Dis Markers. 2014.
- Haneline M, et al. "An analysis of the etiology of cervical artery dissections: 1994-2003." Journal of Manipulative and Physiological Therapeutics.2005;28:617-622.
- Haldeman S, et al. "Clinical perceptions of the risk of vertebral artery dissection after cervical manipulation: the effect of referral bias." Spine.2002;2:334-342.
- "Recognition of Spontaneous Vertebral Artery Dissection Preempting Spinal Manipulative Therapy: A Patient Presenting With Neck Pain and Headache for Chiropractic Care" by Mattox et al. and published in the Journal of Chiropractic Medicine (June 2014)
- "Risk of Vertebrobasilar Stroke and Chiropractic Care" by Cassidy et. al. and published in the journal Spine (February 2008)

- "Changes in Vertebral Artery Blood Flow Following Various Head Positions and Cervical Spine Manipulation" by Quesnele et. al. and published in JMPT (January 2014)
- "Chiropractic and Stroke: Association or Causation?" by P. Tuchin and published in the International Journal of Clinical Practice (Sept. 2013)
- "Chiropractic Manipulation & Cervical Artery Dissection" by Michael T. Haneline, DC, MPH, and Gary Lewkovich, DC, and published in JACA (January/February 2007)
- "Internal Forces Sustained by the Vertebral Artery During Spinal Manipulative Therapy" by Bruce P. Symons, DC, Tim Leonard, and Walter Herzog, PhD, and published in JMPT (October 2002)
- "Cervical Manipulation and the Myth of Stroke" by Donald Murphy, DC, DACAN, and published in Medicine & Health (June 2012)
- The following information was taken from the American Chiropractic Association's website.

Benefits and Risks of Neck Pain Treatments

Neck pain will affect about 70% of the population at some point in their lives and is a common reason many individuals seek help from a health care professional. A particular episode of neck-related problems can be mildly irritating, or it could be seriously debilitating.

While recent scientific studies have found that there are useful treatments for many neck-related problems, no one treatment has been shown to be effective in all cases. Commonly used physical treatments for neck pain include spinal manipulation, mobilization, massage, and therapeutic exercises. Common pharmaceutical treatments include acetaminophen, non-steroidal anti-inflammatory drugs (NSAIDs), muscle relaxant medications, and narcotic (opioid) pain medications.

All of the commonly used neck pain treatments carry some risk. Most of these risks are mild, but some can be serious.

To outline the benefits and relative risks of these therapies, the American Chiropractic Association (ACA) has prepared this summary of recent scientific findings. This review includes information from a report of the Bone and Joint Decade 2000-2010 Task Force on Neck Pain and Its Associated Disorders[65].

This international, multi- disciplinary team of researchers examined available research studies to determine the best treatments for neck pain. This summary also includes another recent review of the scientific evidence on the potential harms and efficacy of commonly used therapies for neck pain[66]. Additional research that describes the efficacy and risks (serious and non- serious) related to these therapies is also reviewed.

Physical Treatments: Manipulation, Mobilization, Massage and Exercise

Manipulation is a therapy in which a trained professional uses his/her hands to gently and quickly move abnormally stiff joints into their normal functional range of motion. Mobilization technique is similar, but it is usually performed more slowly.

Evidence from numerous clinical studies has shown that both manipulation and mobilization of the cervical spine (the neck) result in short-term improvements in pain and physical function, as well as lasting, long-term pain relief. The report by the Bone and Joint Decade Task Force on Neck Pain and Its Associated Disorders, referenced above, found 17 studies that looked at various manual therapies. It found overall positive evidence for both mobilization and manipulation, particularly when combined with exercise. This led the authors to include mobilization, manipulation and other manual therapies among the "likely helpful" treatments for simple neck pain.

A variety of minor side effects are commonly reported with all manual treatments for neck pain. These include temporary aggravations in symptoms or mild/moderate soreness following manipulation, mobilization, massage, or therapeutic exercises of the cervical spine.

The relation between manual treatments and serious complications is controversial. Numerous case reports have associated cervical spine manipulation with a rare type of stroke that results from a dissection (tear) of the vertebral artery, a blood vessel in the neck. These dissections are likely due to an underlying abnormality of the vascular system that usually can't be identified in advance, and are probably not directly caused by the manipulation. Unfortunately, the only early sign of an evolving dissection is neck pain and headache, symptoms that may lead people to seek treatment from a doctor of chiropractic or other professional.

The largest study performed to date looked at the medical records of 11 million people in the Canadian Provence of Ontario over a nine year period and found that patients who went to a doctor of chiropractic for neck pain were no more likely to have a stroke following a chiropractic visit than patients who went to their primary care medical physician for neck pain[67].

That study concluded that any observed association between a stroke and a patient's visit to either a chiropractic physician or a family medical physician was not directly caused by any treatment performed. Instead, any association was likely due to patients with an evolving vertebral artery dissection seeking care for symptoms such as neck pain or headache that sometimes take place before the stroke occurs.

The likelihood of a person having one of these rare vertebral artery strokes is about 1 to 3 per 100,000 people and is similar among both chiropractic patients and the general population.

Pharmaceutical Treatments: Acetaminophen, NSAIDs, Muscle Relaxant Medications and Narcotics

Simple analgesics such as acetaminophen (paracetamol) are commonly used to treat neck-related conditions. While generally safe at recommended doses, acetaminophen is the largest cause of drug overdoses in the United States because of the narrow range between therapeutic dose and toxic dose[68]. Every year in the United States, acetaminophen overdoses are responsible for 56,000 emergency room visits, 2,600 hospitalizations, and 458 deaths due to acute liver failure.

NSAIDs are often used to treat neck-related conditions. Common side effects include nausea, vomiting, and abdominal pain. NSAID use has been associated with a variety of serious adverse effects including bleeding and ulcers in the stomach and intestine, stroke, kidney failure, life-threatening allergic reactions, and liver failure. One study published in The New England Journal of Medicine[69] estimated that at least 103,000 patients are hospitalized per year in the United States for serious gastrointestinal complications due to NSAID use. These authors also estimated that there are 16,500 NSAID-related deaths annually in the United States, making this the 15th most common cause of death. This figure is similar to the annual number of deaths from AIDS, and is considerably greater than the number of deaths from multiple myeloma, asthma, or cervical cancer.

NSAIDs also can have significant cardiovascular side effects. One recent review[70] found that major vascular complications were increased by about a third in patients taking one of the "new generation" coxib NSAIDs. It also found that ibuprofen significantly increased major coronary events. This study found that among 1,000 patients taking a coxib or diclofenac for a year, one would expect three more major vascular events and one additional fatality, compared with placebo.

Skeletal muscle relaxant drugs including benzodiazepines such as Diazepam (Valium®) are often used for treatment of neck pain. The most commonly reported side effects are drowsiness, fatigue, and muscle weakness. Less common side effects include confusion, depression, vertigo, constipation, blurred vision, and amnesia[71].

The use of narcotic (opioid) pain medications frequently leads to nausea, vomiting, constipation, and dizziness. Both muscle relaxants and narcotic pain medications produce drowsiness that may impair working or driving in about 1 in 3 patients. Muscle relaxants and narcotics are associated with significant risk of abuse, addiction, dependence, withdrawal, seizures, potentially fatal injuries to the liver, and potentially fatal overdoses. Overdoses of opioid painkillers are responsible for some 15,000 deaths per year, more than the number of deaths from cocaine and heroin combined[72].

Comparative Effectiveness of Common Treatments
One review article concluded that there is moderate- to high-quality evidence that patients with some types of chronic neck pain have clinically important short-term and long-term improvements from a course of spinal manipulation or mobilization, but similar benefits were not seen from massage.

One recent study[73] compared three groups of neck pain patients who were treated with
1) spinal manipulation,
2) an exercise program, or
3) medications, including NSAIDs, acetaminophen, or (in non-responsive patients) narcotic medications and/or muscle relaxants.

This study found that the patients who were treated with either spinal manipulation or the exercise program had significantly greater relief of pain in the short term and in the long term (up to one year after treatment ended).

The Bone and Joint Decade Task Force review[65] concluded that therapies that were "likely helpful" for non- traumatic neck pain included manipulation, mobilization, and exercises. They concluded that there was "not enough evidence to make a determination" about the helpfulness of NSAIDs and other drugs.

Conclusion

The current scientific evidence indicates that all commonly used treatments for neck pain have limited evidence of effectiveness. All treatments come with fairly common but mild side effects, and some have rare but potentially serious side effects. In general, the physical treatments (including manipulation, mobilization, massage and exercise) have fairly good evidence of effectiveness and are very rarely associated with any serious complications. Pharmaceutical treatments, although commonly used, have limited evidence of effectiveness for treatment of neck pain, and infrequent but potentially serious complications.

In conclusion, there is good epidemiological evidence that the odds of having a stroke following a visit to a doctor of chiropractic are no greater than the odds of having a stroke following a visit to a primary care doctor[67]. In addition, there is biomechanical evidence that cervical manipulation stretches the vertebral arteries less than routine examination procedures[74], making it unlikely that a cervical manipulation can physically cause an arterial dissection. There is evidence that a manual approach to neck pain including manipulation is at least as effective as a conventional approach using NSAIDs and/or opiates with no greater risk of complications.

Neck pain patients who do not present with signs or symptoms of serious underlying disease should be given the choice of whether to pursue manual treatments, pharmaceutical treatments, or a combination of both. Shared decision-making should be based on complete and unbiased information, and patient preference should be respected.

Jeff S. Williams, DC, FIANM

CHIROPRACTIC CERVICAL MANIPULATION: PUTTING BENEFITS & RISKS INTO PROPER PERSPECTIVE

From the start, let me state that research simply does **NOT** support the "Chiropractors Cause Strokes" myth.

Through the **RAND** Institute, it is estimated that a **serious**, adverse reaction (such as stroke as a result to a chiropractic adjustment alone) happens in approximately 1 out of every 1 million treatments. Keep in mind the "**1 out of every 1-2 million**" number as you read through this article.

Let's put that finding into perspective by comparing it to some other odds.
- The odds of being struck and killed by lightning is **1 in 174,426** according to the National Safety Council.
- The odds of being told to "Come on down," on The Price Is Right is **1 in 36!**
- The odds of being born with 11 fingers or toes is **1 in 500.**
- The odds of dying from a firearms assault is **1 in 113.**
- How about this one: the odds of winning an Oscar are **1 in 11,500.**

LOOKS LIKE IT'S TIME TO MOVE TO LA!

Let's pack up the truck and move to Beverly!

The simple message is that there is very little (to zero) risk at all of a chiropractic adjustment being the **lone** cause of a person having suffered a stroke.

If Doctors of Chiropractic were out in the world causing strokes "all of the time," it would be apparent, it would be obvious, and our malpractice insurance would reflect the fact that a visit to the chiropractor comes with a considerable amount of risk.

To the contrary, we chiropractors have malpractice insurance that costs approximately 1/10th of what it costs our medical counterparts.

Before we start diving off into the research too deeply, I want to talk about a case that happened within the last couple of years (February 2016) that brought the "Chiropractors Cause Strokes" myth back to the forefront. It had to do with the **"Queen of Snapchat," Katie May.**

Katie died of a stroke at the age of 34 and, by many, it was immediately assumed the stroke was a result of her two visits to a chiropractor to treat her recent onset of neck pain.

I actually wrote about this case shortly after it originally happened. Initial reports stated that she had a horrible fall while on the set of a photo shoot, which resulted in her neck pain. Then, for some reason, this fact seemed to disappear from further reports.

In addition, initial reports stated that Katie visited either the ER or a medical professional prior to her visits with a chiropractor. The family later denied this so, admittedly, there is some confusion on the matter. Certainly when you consider the family is now suing the chiropractor.

Considering this information, let's begin breaking it all down.

Katie posted this message to Twitter: *"Pinched a nerve in my neck **on a photo shoot** and got adjusted this morning. It really hurts! Any home remedy suggestions loves? XOXO."*

Keep that in mind as we run through things that can cause a vertebral artery dissection like Katie May suffered. They are as follows:
- **Physical Trauma (direct blow to the neck,** traffic collision, etc.)
- Strangulation
- Spontaneous (from underlying connective tissue disorder)

According to a paper by Debette et. al., "Trauma has been reported to have occurred within a month of dissection in 40% with nearly **90% of this time the trauma being minor[75].** "

Vertebral artery dissection (VAD) can be particularly difficult to diagnose without the use of a CT Angiogram. For instance, some common symptoms of VAD are as follows:

- Pain and/or numbness in the same side of the face.
- Head pain/Headache that develops gradually and can be dull or throbbing
- In less than 1/5thof the cases of VAD, people suffer difficulty speaking or swallowing.
- Possible unsteadiness or lack of coordination
- Visual abnormalities
- Hiccups
- Nausea/Vomiting
- Hearing loss

When one reads this list, it seems easy to diagnose a VAD, right?

The problem lies in the fact that VAD rarely presents with these classic signs. VAD commonly presents as a healthy patient that shows up with a headache or neck pain and sometimes both. In fact, it is estimated that more than 80% of VAD cases present with neck pain and headache alone.

Is a medical professional or chiropractor going to refer **every single one** of these patients for a CT Angiogram or an MRI?

NOT VERY LIKELY.

It is simply not economically feasible to do so and good luck getting insurance companies to cover the costs on all of those CT Angiograms and MRIs!

If Katie did indeed visit a medical professional after her fall, they missed it. Unfortunately, it seems that the chiropractor missed it as well. That does not, however, mean the two professionals are inept. As the website for **emedicine.com** states, "The focal signs may not appear until after a latent period lasting as long as three days, however, and **delays of weeks and years also have been reported[76]**."

That being said, I don't want to be completely biased here. If a healthy person shows up with a headache and neck pain **BUT** has a history of recent trauma, more exploration is advised, without question. Knowing this, I can relay **countless** stories of medical doctors having made bad decisions as well. I have heard many stories throughout my twenty years of practice. A study that we will discuss later shows that people commonly present to a chiropractor or a primary practitioner (medical doctor) already suffering an artery dissection before even walking into the office and assuming the pain is a result of something innocent and simple. This is one example of why chiropractors and medical doctors both carry malpractice insurance.

But, as I mentioned before, chiropractors' malpractice is approximately 1/10th the cost of their medical counterparts because, basically, **we chiropractors do not typically cause harms in our patients. Malpractice carriers have done their homework and it is clear that there is little to zero risk in going to a chiropractor.**

As we go through more and more papers, it should be clear that Katie likely suffered the VAD as a result of the fall during the photo shoot and the VAD was missed by the medical professionals (if she did indeed go) and then certainly missed by the chiropractor **BUT**, the chiropractor almost certainly did not **CAUSE** the VAD. There's no way he helped it, and he could have even potentially exacerbated it. But it is highly doubtful and exceedingly rare that he could have been the lone **CAUSE** of it.

Sometime later, the Los Angeles coroner reported that the chiropractor was the one responsible for Katie's death. This finding opened the door wide to all of the chiropractic haters to bash away at the profession. Chiropractrors cause strokes....right?

The LA coroner's office is an appointed position that, in some states, requires little training, to be quite honest. While I am unaware of this particular coroner's level of training and expertise, this coroner has been under scrutiny for being understaffed and underfunded to mention just a couple of issues. In addition, I would argue that simply because a man or a woman is a county coroner does not mean they are above being affected by bias or by their profession's long-held beliefs and teachings. I would say they most certainly are not above influence and, in my opinion, are actually highly likely to be affected.

I would also argue that the coroner likely has little to **zero** knowledge of the current body of research regarding cervical manipulation and the instance of stroke. How could an educated person aware of the body of literature on the matter make a definitive judgment such as this?

For years, I have experienced nurses, physician assistants, medical doctors, and others in an online setting claiming that chiropractic adjustments are dangerous and ineffective. They claim that commonly, chiropractors cause strokes. A theme amongst them is, **"It happens all of the time."** We see it **"all of the time."**

RESEARCH SUGGESTS THAT NOTION IS A LIE.

Or, at minimum, it is ignorance and misunderstanding of their experiences.

To put it in plain and simple terms, these detractors wonder why someone would undergo a treatment that is so dangerous for absolutely no improvement. That is in their understanding and in their opinion, of course. Again, this simply shows ignorance in regard to the available research. I would like to be less dramatic or inflammatory in my wording but I don't know any other way to describe it.

Let's assume for a moment that this "Chiropractors Cause Strokes" myth has its base rooted in some sort of fact. Let us be clear. **It does not.** But, for argument sake, let us say that it does. At that point, we would need to assess the **benefits** of chiropractic treatment vs. the **risks** of chiropractic treatment.

In Southern terms, "Is the squeeze worth the push?"

IS THERE A RETURN ON THE INVESTMENT?

Again, this is purely for argument sake because the "Chiropractors Cause Strokes" myth is not real to start with but playing the devil's advocate can be of use and is almost always entertaining.

Before we step into deeper waters with the research papers, let us discuss **benefits & effectiveness vs. risk for some common treatments for spinal complaints in the medical world.** If the discussion is focused on doing away with cervical adjustments, what then would be the alternatives and how effective are they?

Basically, if the medical field is looking into OUR backyard, maybe we should take a peek into theirs as well.

IT IS ONLY FAIR.

- The opioid crisis cost the US economy $504 billion dollars in 2015and a total of $221 billion to $431 billion in lost economic output due to there being 33,000 opioid-related deaths in 2015 [77]
- "There were 63,600 opioid-related deaths in 2016, which was an increase of 21% from the 2015[78]"
- Chou R, et. al. – "Although the steroid injections for radiculopathy showed some short-term relief in pain and short-term increase in function, the benefits seen in

Jeff S. Williams, DC, FIANM

the patients were only small and short-term only. There was no effect long-term and no affect on whether or not the person had surgery eventually. The evidence in this paper suggested there was no effectiveness at all for the treatment of spinal stenosis[32]"

- Epstein N, et. al. – "Although not approved by the Food and Drug Administration (FDA), injections are being performed with an increased frequency (160%), are typically short-acting and ineffective over the longer-term, while exposing patients to major risks/complications[79]"

- Peterson CK, et. al. – "Subacute/chronic patients treated with SMT (spinal manipulative therapy) were significantly more likely to report relevant "improvement" compared with CNRI (CERVICAL NERVE ROOT INJECTION) patients. There was no difference in outcomes when comparing acute patients only[28]"

- Chou R, et. al. – "Epidural corticosteroid injections for radiculopathy were associated with immediate improvements in pain and might be associated with immediate improvements in function, but benefits were small and not sustained, and there was no effect on long-term risk of surgery. Evidence did not suggest that effectiveness varies based on injection technique, corticosteroid, dose, or comparator. Limited evidence suggested that epidural corticosteroid injections are not effective for spinal stenosis or non-radicular back pain and that facet joint corticosteroid injections are not effective for presumed facet joint pain[39]."

- Chou R, et. al – "Surgery for radiculopathy with herniated lumbar disc and symptomatic spinal stenosis is associated with short-term benefits compared to nonsurgical therapy, though benefits diminish with long-term follow-up in some trials. For non-radicular back pain with common degenerative changes, fusion is no more effective than intensive rehabilitation, but associated with small to moderate benefits compared to standard nonsurgical therapy[39]."

- Maghout J, et. al. – "Use of intervertebral fusion devices rose rapidly after their introduction in 1996. This increased use was associated with an increased complication risk without improving disability or re-operation rates[42]."

At this point, it is clear the medical field has its own issues to concentrate and improve upon when it comes to spinal pain and its treatment. Imagine the progress they could achieve without concentrating so much effort against the chiropractic community!

Chiropractic as a pseudo-science:

I think most people are reasonable. They understand that chiropractic was first discovered, or proposed, as a treatment by D.D. Palmer in the late 1800's and the profession was furthered by his son, BJ. Palmer until his passing in 1961.

Some on the medical end of healthcare will point to the father and son and their assertions as a reason for people to turn away from present-day chiropractic. After all, DD Palmer, as so many others of that time, was searching for new ways of doing things. He was classified in the beginning as a 'magnetic healer'. That makes him an easy target even over 100 years later.

I would say that, as with anything, chiropractic has greatly expanded and advanced in understanding and in what it has to offer as well as in the research that backs the use of spinal manipulation, exercise, and mobilization.

Just think about it, when chiropractic was first made into a healthcare treatment modality, medical doctors were still performing what I call 'The Three L's'; blood letting, leeching, and lobotomies. Let's just keep things in perspective.

To be direct, many chiropractors refer to, and accept referrals from, medical doctors daily. This is not a "doctor of chiropractic vs. medical doctor" discussion at all. The attempt here is not to compare two different professions that both deserve a great deal of respect.

The goal is to educate about the benefits and risks of cervical manipulation and to keep things in proper perspective and context.

Many of chiropractic's detractors have built a life of comfort from their opposition to the profession. They own and operate big websites, write articles and books, and give lectures and seminars opposing chiropractic. I can promise you, regardless of what they say, there will NEVER be enough research that comes out that will make them reconsider and say something like, "You know, my whole life, I was wrong about chiropractic. They weren't the fools. I was the fool. Now, I'd like to re-think everything hateful I've ever said about chiropractic for the last several decades."

This isn't going to happen so, no matter the research quantity or quality that supports chiropractic, they will continue the crusade by calling it rubbish (and all kinds of other names) so that they can continue with their lifestyles and maintain their reputation and "integrity." But, that's OK. As long as you know that most of this research is done by governments, insurance companies, Universities, and medical doctors. These are the people that either don't necessarily have a dog in the hunt or people that simply do not like chiropractors. That is precisely why I feel that you can trust the research.

Let's begin with the benefits of adjustments for the neck in particular.
A 2003 study published in the British Medical Journal concluded that manual therapy (spinal mobilization) is more effective and less costly for treating neck pain than physiotherapy, physical therapy, or care by a general practitioner.

This 2014 study by Dewitte et. al[80]. published in Manual Therapy concluded "Pending on these patterns, specific mobilization and manipulation techniques are warranted. The proposed patterns are illustrated in 3 case studies. This clinical algorithm is the corollary of empirical expertise and is complemented by in-depth discussions and knowledge exchange with international colleagues. Consequently, it is intended that a carefully targeted approach contributes to an increase in specificity and safety in the use of cervical mobilizations and manipulation techniques as valuable adjuncts to other manual therapy modalities."

A 2011 randomized clinical trial by Dunning et. al [81]. published in the Journal Of Orthopedic Sports Physical Therapy concluded "The combination of upper cervical and upper thoracic HVLA thrust manipulation is appreciably more effective in the short term than non-thrust mobilization in patients with mechanical neck pain."

2011 by Yu et. al. [82] concluded "Chiropractic management of atlantoaxial osteoarthritis yielded favorable outcomes for these 10 patients."

2011 Puentedura et. al. [83] published in the Journal of Orthopedic Sports Physical Therapists concluded "Patients with neck pain demonstrated a more favorable response when the (spinal mobilization) was directed to the cervical spine rather than the thoracic spine. Patients receiving cervical (spinal mobilization) also demonstrated fewer transient side-effects."

2008 – Led by J. Guzman[65], The Bone and Joint Decade 2000-2010 Task Force on Neck Pain and Its Associated Disorders published their paper in SPINE journal . It was made up of an international, multi-disciplinary team of researchers that examined available research studies to determine the best treatments for neck pain. They found 17 studies that looked at various manual therapies. It found overall positive evidence for both mobilization and manipulation, particularly when combined with exercise. This led the authors to include mobilization, manipulation and other manual therapies among the "likely helpful" treatments for simple neck pain.

In comparison to anti-inflammatories, they concluded that there was "not enough evidence to make a determination" about the helpfulness of NSAIDs and other drugs.

Now for the benefits in headaches and migraines.

2016 – by Dunning et. al. [81]and published in the BioMed Central Musculoskeletal Disorders journal concluded that Six to eight sessions of upper cervical and upper thoracic manipulation were shown to be more effective than mobilization and exercise in patients with chronic headache, and the effects were maintained at 3 months.

1998 – Nelson, et. al. [36] and published in Journal of Manipulative and Physiological Therapeutics study concluded patients who received only chiropractic care showed significant improvement, on par with those given the powerful prescription drug but without the side effects. The headache index, from a diary kept by each patient, showed chiropractic to have reduced the severity and frequency of headaches as well or better than the combined therapy or amitriptyline alone at each stage of the study.

2000 – A randomized clinical trial by Tuchin et. al. [84] published in Journal of Manipulative and Physiological Therapeutics concluded that the results of this study support previous results showing that some people report significant improvement in migraines after chiropractic. Over 80% of participants reported stress as a major factor for their migraines. It appears probable that chiropractic care has an effect on the physical conditions related to stress and that in these people the effects of the migraine are reduced.

2001 – by Bronfort et. al. [30] This paper concluded that chiropractic appears to have a better effect than massage for cervicogenic headache. It also appears that spinal manipulation has an effect comparable to commonly used first-line prophylactic prescription medications for tension-type headache and migraine headache.

2011 – Duke University[85] published a paper in Spine Journal and said the study adds to the support of chiropractic in moderate doses as a viable option for the treatment of cervicogenic headaches.

Clearly, the benefit has been established time and time again. If someone claims there is no benefit beyond that of simple mobilization, massage, or exercise, then they are ignorant of the information.

Now, again, the complaint among some chiropractic detractors is that there is too much risk for what they claim is no benefit. I have established the benefit. **Now, let's discuss the risk. Or lack thereof.**

2015 – Kosloff et. al. [86] published in Chiropractic and Manual therapies. They state the following: We found no significant association between exposure to chiropractic care and the risk of vertebral artery stroke. We conclude that manipulation is an unlikely cause of vertebral artery stroke. The positive association between primary doctor visits and vertebral artery stroke is most likely due to patient decisions to seek care for the symptoms (headache and neck pain) of arterial dissection.

2015 – Whedon et. al. [35] studied the risk of chiropractic in older patients. Here's what they found: Among Medicare B beneficiaries aged 66 to 99 years with neck pain, the incidence of vertebrobasilar stroke was too low to allow further analysis. Chiropractic cervical spine manipulation is unlikely to cause stroke in patients aged 66 to 99 years with neck pain.

2008 – This one was a big one – Cassidy et.al.[67] did a comprehensive study with 9 years of compiled information. **NINE** years! Vertebral artery stroke is a very rare event in the population. The increased risks of VBA stroke associated with chiropractic and general practitioner visits **is likely due to patients with headache and neck pain from VBA dissection seeking care before their stroke. We found no evidence of excess risk of VBA stroke associated with chiropractic care compared to primary care.**

I hope I have adequately demonstrated through research that the benefits of cervical adjustments are most certainly there and that the risks are extremely low. Let's be clear though. There are risks. There are risks with EVERYTHING you do including walking into the street. However, when we are objective and put things in proper context, it's clear that the risk is minimal compared to the benefits.

Let's do some comparing and contrasting here for the proper perspective. Let's talk about something as innocuous as **acetaminophen**, which is found in Tylenol. Tylenol is responsible for 56,000 emergency room visits per year, 2,600 hospitalizations, and 458 deaths. **PER YEAR.** That's just acetaminophen. Anti-inflammatories all together are estimated to be responsible for 16,500 deaths per year. Once again, let's keep it all in proper perspective.

There are 70,000 chiropractors in the U.S. making Chiropractic the third largest doctoral-level discipline in America, yet Chiropractors have the lowest malpractice costs by a significant margin. The reason is that there is little risk in being treated by a chiropractor. If strokes "happen all of the time," chiropractic malpractice insurance would be sky-high, yet it's the cheapest.

Looking at this graphic provided by the ACA, you can see that it's estimated there are 5-10 complications following adjustments in approximately 10 million or about 1 in 1 million.

As I have said, there are risks with any treatment you can imagine including exercise, yoga, massage, or just taking a Tylenol. But when kept in proper perspective and context, it's clear that chiropractic doesn't carry a risk near any type of treatment in the traditional medical path.

To put the proverbial "period" at the end of the sentence, The Bone and Joint Decade Task Force review concluded that, in general, the physical treatments (including manipulation, mobilization, massage and exercise) have good evidence of effectiveness and are very rarely associated with any serious complications.

As you can tell, this situation has lots of different signs that cross over into other conditions and can be EXTREMELY difficult to recognize for anyone, be it chiropractor or medical doctor - even an emergency room doctor.

Finally, why would there be a faction of the healthcare world that holds such disdain for chiropractic that they would willfully ignore research and propagate lies about the profession?

Let me be honest and make an attempt at being completely objective: it's partly because some chiropractors deserve it.

If I were a medical doctor and I saw a chiropractor saying they can cure cancer, I would have a problem with that. It is easy to understand that many times, those in medical world see and hear the worst of the worst for different conditions.

For example, how many times does someone waltz in talking about how amazing their chiropractor is? It happens but, in general, patients go to their medical doctor to talk about what's WRONG with them. Not about what feels good on account of their chiropractor.

I would also agree that some chiropractors may be particularly aggressive and use rotational maneuvers while others are not aggressive and do not employ rotational maneuvers. Some styles of treatment will certainly put a patient at more risk for stroke.

Now that I've said that, I'll say this: **MOST** of the reason there are certain circles of chiropractic detractors in the medical world can be traced to the American Medical Association. In a case called Wilk vs. AMA, it was proven in Federal Court that the American Medical Association did the following or encouraged their members in the following manner:
- Encourage ethical complaints against doctors of chiropractic;
- Oppose chiropractic inroads in health insurance;
- Oppose chiropractic inroads in workmen's compensation;

Jeff S. Williams, DC, FIANM

- Oppose chiropractic inroads into labor unions;
- Oppose chiropractic inroads into hospitals; and
- Contain chiropractic schools.
- Conducting nationwide conferences on chiropractic;
- Distributing publications critical of chiropractic;
- Assisting others in preparation of anti-chiropractic literature;
- Warning that professional association between medical physicians and chiropractors was unethical; and
- Discouraging colleges, universities and faculty from cooperating with chiropractic schools.

This behavior started in the 1960's and was passed down to all of the state medical associations then down to the individual practitioners in each state. This attack on Chiropractic did not officially end until the 1990's although I'd argue that it is not over.

The AMA lost the case, by the way.

Considering this was proven in Federal Court, it isn't hard to understand (or very surprising) that the anti-chiropractic chants that come about every single time a tragedy occurs, no matter how rare it actually is, will continue.

As long as people are educated to the actual facts, research, and stats, you should be able to keep the discussion and emotions that result from this sort of story in the proper context and perspective.

A methodical, logical, and systematic stroll through the body of literature shows without a doubt there is indeed incredible benefit in the use of cervical manipulative treatments for neck pain and headaches & migraine complaints while there is no more risk of stroke from treating with a chiropractor vs. treating with a medical professional.

I want this article to be the final word on this "Chiropractors Cause Strokes" myth. I want it to be the "end all, be all" on the topic but I have lived long enough to know better and have experienced twenty years within the chiropractic profession. I know this information will not change the attitudes of many. But, if this article can be a reference point for learning more about the topic and can be a tool for educating others about this myth, then I will have fulfilled my function.

In conclusion, the benefit and effectiveness has been proven, the risks have been disproved, and the "Chiropractors Cause Strokes" myth is ONCE AND FOR ALL officially and completely DEBUNKED.

RISK FROM CHIROPRACTIC ADJUSTMENT SAME AS VISIT WITH MEDICAL DOCTOR

Why They Did It
With periodic accusations as to the supposed relationship between stroke and chiropractic manipulation, researchers are consistently interested in further exploration and understanding on the topic. The authors of this paper wanted to compare stroke as a consequence of having had a chiropractic visit and the incidence of stroke as a consequence of a primary care physician visit.

How They Did It
- The study was case controlled
- Involved those on the Medicare advantage plan
- The study accepted subjects from January 1, 2011 and December 31, 2013
- Several different parameters were considered in the analysis of the data.

What They Found
- Between that time. There were 1829 vertebral artery stroke cases
- No association was found between chiropractic visits and vertebral artery stroke period

- Also, there was no association between primary care physician visits and vertebral artery strokes period
- Also worthy of note, the findings showed chiropractic visits did not even Report manipulation occurring in almost one third of the strokes period

Wrap It Up

The authors of the paper concluded chiropractic manipulation is an unlikely cause of vertebral artery stroke.

As the Cassidy study showed over a course of nine years, there is no greater risk in undergoing chiropractic manipulation than if one goes to a primary care physician.

Essentially, people are visiting both healthcare professionals suffering symptoms that are most likely originating from the vertebral artery stroke already in progress[86].

HAVE YOU EVERY HAD SOMEONE TELL YOU CHIROPRACTORS ARE DANGEROUS?

Why They Did It

The authors of this paper were focused on what kind of changes, if any, are present within the vertebral arteries of the neck when a cervical adjustment is performed by a chiropractor or when placed in various positions.

How They Did It

- This paper was done as a blinded examiner cohort study involving four randomized clinical tasks.
- 10 males (24-30 yrs old) were the test subjects.
- None of the test subjects had significant health history within the last six months.
- Measurements were taken at the C1 and C2 spinal level in the normal, neutral position.

- The subjects were placed in 3 different positions as well as having had Chiropractic upper cervical adjustments.
- MRI technology was used to collect accurate information in the different positions as well as during the chiropractic spinal manipulation.
- Differences in the flow and velocity of the vertebral arteries were performed via repeated measures analysis of variance.

What They Found

There were no significant differences, when compared from side to side, for flow or velocity.

Wrap It Up

"There were no significant changes in blood flow or velocity in the vertebral arteries of healthy young male adults after various head positions and cervical spine manipulations[87]."

RESEARCH TO KNOW ABOUT CHIROPRACTORS AND SAFETY

Why They Did It

The authors of this paper wanted to explore the potential for injury or damage from a chiropractic adjustment of the C1 on C2 (atlanto-axial) segment, also known as a high velocity/low amplitude (HVLA) thrust. They noticed the literature is completely lacking in this aspect, and they hoped to fill the gaps in knowledge. Knowing the exact mechanisms and forces involved helps further understanding of the treatment.

How They Did It

- The authors employed an ultrasound motion tracking mechanism called the Zebris CMS20.

Jeff S. Williams, DC, FIANM

- 20 human subjects were accepted for use in the study.
- The placement and interaction of C1 on C2 was analyzed with three HVLA movements into rotation.

What They Found
- The mean norm of displacement during the movement was 0.5mm.
- The maximum displacement during the movements was 6mm.
- Displacement factors were not reproducible.

Wrap It Up
The authors of this paper concluded the following, "Displacement during the execution of HVLA thrust is unintentional, unpredictable, and not reproducible. On the other hand and in accordance with other studies, the displacement induced with the present technique seems not to be able to endanger vital structure on the Spinal Cord and the Vertebral Artery[88]."

HOW SAFE IS A CHIROPRACTIC ADJUSTMENT?

Unfortunately, there is more than enough misinformation in the world about the safety of chiropractic adjustments. Any chiropractor you speak with will have plenty of stories to tell in which a provider in the medical field told one of their patients that chiropractors will hurt or even kill them. It is, unfortunately, incredibly common and profoundly disappointing.

I had a patient share with me just last week that she expressed her plan to take her father to see me. Her father's doctor was very adamant, and even a bit scolding, when he said, "They will kill you. They will absolutely kill your dad."

Let's be fair here; I truly believe this opinion came from a place of caring for their patient. However, it also came from an incredible amount of ignorance of what chiropractors do and how they do it. Not to mention how safe what chiropractors do is. Many in the medical field know nothing at all of the different techniques and different protocols used in the profession.

This ignorance originates from either anti-chiropractic dogma that has been passed down from the American Medical Association or from the simple laziness required to avoid and ignore educating themselves about other forms of treatment for neuromusculoskeletal conditions. They have not educated themselves on alternative means of treating outside of medications and the research behind them. Let's face it; the medical field has only treated non-complicated neuromusculoskeletal conditions with pills until recently. It is not something that they know much about.

Here is a paper having to do with assessing damage from spinal manipulation.

Why They Did It

The authors wanted to assess whether there is damage as a result of spinal manipulation and attempt to understand the overall safety of the procedure.

How They Did It
- 30 subjects were accepted for the study.
- They were separated into different study groups
  - Placebo
  - Single lower neck manipulation
  - Thoracic (mid-back) manipulation
- Blood samples were collected prior to the procedure as well as immediately afterward and 2 hours post-procedure.
- The samples were tested for several common "tissue damage" markers such as troponin and creatine phosphokinase to mention a couple.

What They Found

There were no significant markers found as a result of the Chiropractic adjustments.

Wrap It Up

"Our data suggest that the mechanical strain produced by SM seems to be innocuous to the joints and surrounding tissues in healthy subjects[89]."

ARE THEY BEING HONEST IF THEY SAY CHIROPRACTORS ARE DANGEROUS?

Why They Did it

More research against a causal relationship between chiropractic treatment and stroke.

For the purposes of this paper, stroke will be referred to as cervical artery dissection or CAD. The goal here was to perform a systematic review and meta-analysis of the data to further understanding on the subject.

How They Did It
- Relevant search terms were used.
- Each article was reviewed by authors of this paper.
- The papers were graded independently.
- Once accepted, the papers were compiled in a meta-analysis.
- There were 253 articles used.
- The information was then quantified by the GRADE method.

What They Found

The undertaking suggested a small association however, the GRADE system suggests the quality of the evidence to be "very low."

"Our analysis shows a small association between chiropractic neck manipulation and cervical artery dissection. This relationship may be explained by the high risk of bias and confounding in the available studies, and in particular by the known association of neck pain with CAD and with chiropractic manipulation. There is no convincing evidence to support a causal link between chiropractic manipulation and CAD. Belief in a causal link may have significant negative consequences such as numerous episodes of litigation[90]."

ISN'T GOING TO THE CHIROPRACTOR RISKY?

As previously mentioned, although the plight of the chiropractor has improved over the last 5-10 years, it is still not rare to hear things like, "I wouldn't go to a chiropractor. They'll twist your head off." Or something along the lines of, "My family doctor told me to never go to a chiropractor. They'll hurt you." This kind of talk comes from the general public as well as uneducated medical professionals.

The publication date of this paper was February 15, 2015 in Spine journal. Spine journal sounds a bit like a chiropractic publication but it is not. It is for neurologist, orthopedic surgeons, and everyone else concerned with issues of the spine.

Why They Did It

The researchers felt that there was inadequate study into the risk of physical injury from spinal manipulation in older folks (a population at increased risk of any sort of injury) following visits to a Doctor of Chiropractic vs. a visit to their primary care physician.

How They Did It
- Medicare data was analyzed on patients aged 66-99
- All patients had a visit in 2007 for a neuromusculoskeletal complaint.
- Using standardized testing, the patients were evaluated within 7 days.
- They compared those treated by a Doctor of Chiropractic against those evaluated by a primary care physician.

What They Found
- The risk for injury in the chiropractic group was lower than that of the primary care group.
- The cumulative probability of injury in the primary care physician group was 153 per 100,000 subjects.
- The cumulative probability of injury in the chiropractic group was 40 injuries per 100,000 subjects.

Wrap It Up
"Among Medicare beneficiaries aged 66-99 with an office visit risk for a neuromusculoskeletal problem, risk of injury to the head, neck, or trunk within 7 days was 76% lower among subjects with a chiropractic office visit than among those who saw a primary care physician[35]."

CERVICAL CURVATURE STUDIES

I chose to include this section due to techniques used by many chiropractors. For some, they have been taught that a decrease in cervical curvature can lead to dire consequences years in the future. They have typically been taught this by practice management companies and sometimes they have even been taught the idea by professors in their chiropractic colleges.

A common treatment protocol using cervical curvature correction as the focus (and practice management technique) may include periodic x-rays throughout treatment. This is not recommended by current research and guidelines.

Another common trait of this type of practice includes recommendations for 50-70 plus visits in a year. Again, this is not usually recommended by current chiropractic research and guidelines.

In some practices, the clinic even requires the patients sign treatment contracts for reduced cost of treatment and hold the threat of collecting on the discount should a patient opt out of treatment. This has become such an unethical problem that many states have made the practice illegal.

My point in including these studies here is to present an argument against the use of cervical curvature as a practice-building technique based on the chiropractic research literature and to bring evidence-based practitioners closer to a truly patient-centered approach to treatment protocols.

There is an argument to be made that degenerative changes and cervical hypolordosis could potentially have some impact in some unknown manner. However, the argument being made herein is that, according to current research, whatever impact it might have appears minimal and certainly not on the level of basing an evidence-based practice on the impact, thereby demanding thousands of dollars from patients, hours in treatment time, and the increased stress and anxiety a patient suffers when told they are in danger from a lack of curvature in their neck.

Basically, loss of curve in the neck appears to be of little to no issue. Therefore, it is not advisable to make it an issue or base treatment protocols around it.

With that, let us look some relevant research findings.

A 20-YEAR STUDY

"Twenty-year Longitudinal Follow-up MRI Study of Asymptomatic Volunteers: The Impact of Cervical Alignment on Disk Degeneration," by Okada et. al.[91] and published in Clinical Spine Surgery in December of 2018.

Why They Did It
The authors wanted to evaluate the long-term effect of sagittal alignment of the cervical spine on intervertebral disk degeneration in healthy asymptomatic subjects.

How They Did It
- This study continues a previous 10-year longitudinal study to determine whether sagittal alignment affects disk degeneration during normal aging.

Jeff S. Williams, DC, FIANM

- They assessed 90 healthy subjects (30 men and 60 women) from among 497 volunteers who underwent magnetic resonance imaging (MRI) and plain radiographs of the cervical spine between 1994 and 1996 (follow-up rate 18.1%).
- They compared initial MRIs and follow-up MRIs, conducted at an average of 21.6 years after the initial study
- Subjects were grouped by age at follow-up (under 40 vs. 40 y and older) and by a lordotic or non-lordotic cervical sagittal alignment at baseline.
- They assessed neck pain, stiff shoulders, and upper-arm numbness at follow-up, and examined associations between clinical symptoms and MRI parameters.

What They Found
Nonlordotic cervical alignment was related to the progression of disk degeneration at C7-T1 but not other levels. **Cervical alignment did not affect the development of clinical symptoms in healthy subjects.**

ANOTHER 20-YEAR STUDY

"A 20-year prospective longitudinal MRI study on cervical spine after whiplash injury: Follow-up of a cross-sectional study" by Daimon et. al.[92] published in Journal of Orthopaedic Science in July 2019.

Why They Did It
Some patients suffer from long-lasting symptoms after whiplash injury. However, there are few reports on the long-term changes in the cervical spine after whiplash injury using imaging tests. The purpose of this longitudinal study was to determine the changes on MRI of the cervical spine 20 years after whiplash injury, and to examine the relationships between changes in the cervical spine on MRI and changes in related clinical symptoms.

How They Did It
- 81 subjects participated
- The mean follow-up duration was 21.7 years
- Statistic analyses were used to investigate whether the progression of each MRI finding was associated with the severity of neck pain, stiff shoulders, dizziness, and tinnitus.

What They Found
Progression in the severity of neck pain, stiff shoulders, dizziness, and tinnitus over 20 years were not significantly associated with the progression of degenerative changes in the cervical spine on MRI.

Wrap It Up
Twenty years after whiplash injury, 95% of the subjects showed a progression of degeneration in the cervical spine. The progression of the intervertebral disc degeneration in the cervical spine on MRI after whiplash injury was not significantly associated with changes in the severity of related clinical symptoms, indicating that the degenerative changes on MRI may reflect the physiological aging process rather than post-traumatic sequelae.

SOMETIMES YOU DON'T KNOW

"Loss of cervical lordosis: What is the prognosis?" by Lippa et. al[93]. and published in the Journal of Craniovertebral Junction and Spine in 2017.

Why They Did It
- Faced with the fact that neck pain can have such a big impact on activities of daily living for some and the fact that imaging commonly demonstrated no findings other than hypolordosis, the researchers wanted to answer the questions:

Jeff S. Williams, DC, FIANM

- To which extent such a finding plays a role in the patient's symptoms?
- If it does, what is the role of conservative or even invasive treatment?
- What are the implications for surgery either for decompressive procedures or corrective procedures?

How They Did It

This paper was a narrative review of the most relevant literature on the topic. Papers examined span from the initial epidemiologic reports out of the pre-MRI and computerized tomography era up to the most recent discussions on cervical sagittal alignment and its implications both for the surgical and nonsurgical patient.

What They Found

"The possibility to correlate clinical outcome with alignment of the spinal column seems appealing but is, however, not as easily translatable into practice as it might seem." "…. it is surely difficult to find definite answers considering that pain as a biopsychosocial phenomenon is probably too vast a problem to be simply reduced to any kind of measures, no matter how sophisticated and appealing such a computation may be.

WE CAN LOSE THE CURVE, BUT THAT'S OK

"Cervical lordosis in asymptomatic individuals: a meta-analysis" by Guo et. al[94] and published in the Journal of Orthopedic Surgery and Research in 2018.

Why They Did It

Cervical lordosis has important clinical and surgical implications. Cervical spine curvature is reported with considerable variability in individual studies. The aim of this study was to examine the existence and extent of cervical lordosis in asymptomatic individuals and to evaluate its relationship with age and gender.

How They Did It

- A comprehensive literature search was conducted in several electronic databases
- Random effects meta-analyses were performed to estimate the proportion of asymptomatic individuals with lordosis and the effect size of cervical lordotic curvature in these individuals which followed metaregression analysis to examine the factors affecting cervical lordosis
- Data from 21 studies were used in the study.
- 15,364 asymptomatic individuals, age 42.30 years

What They Found

- 64% individuals possessed lordotic curvature
- Degree of lordotic curvature differed by method of measurement
- Lordotic curvature was not significantly different between symptomatic and asymptomatic individuals but was significantly higher in males in comparison with females
- Age was not significantly associated with lordotic cervical curvature

Wrap It Up

Majority of the asymptomatic individuals possesses lordotic cervical curvature which is higher in males than in females but have no relationship with age or symptoms.

Jeff S. Williams, DC, FIANM

"**Chiropractic conservatism and the ability to determine contra-indications, non-indications, and indications to chiropractic care: a cross-sectional survey of chiropractic students**" by Guillaume Goncalves, Marine Demorier, and et. al[95]. It was published in BMC Chiropractic and Manual Therapies in 2019.

In the background section of the abstract, they start by saying "While there is a broad spectrum of practice within chiropractic two sub-types can be identified, those who focus on musculoskeletal problems and those who treat also non-musculoskeletal problems. The latter group may adhere to the old conservative 'subluxation' model.

The main goal of this study is to determine if chiropractic students with such conservative opinions are likely to have a different approach to determine *contra-indications, non-indications* and *indications* to chiropractic treatment versus those without such opinions."

What They Found
- They had 359 students respond out of 536.
- They generally recognized a number of contra-indication as well as indications for treatment
- What the problem was in identifying non-indications for treatment.
- The subluxation students were much more willing to treat someone even when there was nothing relevant wrong
- For example, they were much more willing to treat a 5-yr-old kid with no history of back pain or disease to prevent future back pain and to also prevent non-musculoskeletal disease.

Wrap Up

Their conclusion was "It is concerning that students who adhere to the subluxation model are prepared to 'operationalize' their conservative opinions in their future scope of practice; apparently willing to treat asymptomatic people with chiropractic adjustments. The determinants of this phenomenon need to be understood."

STUDIES RELATED TO HEADACHES, MIGRAINES, ETC.

AN EXPERT REPORT ABOUT HEADACHES, MASSAGE, AND MANUAL THERAPY

In some circles of the healthcare world, there has remained a controversy about how effective therapies like spinal manipulation (chiropractic) or manual therapy can be in the treatment of headaches. This controversy is specifically related to tension-type headaches.

Those of us that have been treating headaches, neck pain, back pain, and musculoskeletal issues for years using these treatment protocols know that there really is no controversy. I have seen migraines that have been persistent and life-altering for decades disappear after just a week or two of treatment.

If I am honest, I will admit that it about knocked me out the first time or two. Now, I have come to expect it and am actually surprised and shocked if a headache or migraine DOES NOT go away after some consistent treatment.

Again, it is no surprise to us, but that is just anecdotal and the proof of research is always needed when you are aiming to truly make a difference in a very stubborn and "slow-to-adopt-new-ideas" medical industry.

In that spirit, let's take a look at this research paper.

Why They Did It

The authors wanted to try to assess how people suffering from tension-type headaches would respond, on average, to manual therapy techniques.

How They Did It

- There were four groups that the participants were split into.
- The four groups were as follows:
    - suboccipital inhibitory pressure
    - suboccipital spinal manipulation
    - a combination of the two
    - control group
- The SF-12 Questionnaire was used to assess the quality of life and was taken at the beginning of treatment to obtain a starting baseline score. It was also taken at the end of treatment and was again taken a full month following the end of the treatment protocol.
- The patients underwent a four-week treatment protocol.

What They Found

- The suboccipital inhibition group had a significant improvement.
- All groups, except for the control group, improved in regards to pain, physical, and social functioning.
- The combined group showed "improved vitality" and the two treatments involving manipulation also had improved "mental health."

Wrap It Up

"All three treatments were effective at changing different dimensions of quality of life, but the combined treatment showed the most change. The results support the effectiveness of treatments applied to the suboccipital region for patients with tension-type headaches[96]."

Jeff S. Williams, DC, FIANM

RESEARCH PROVES CHIROPRACTIC IS GREAT FOR MIGRAINES

Why They Did It

The stated reasoning for this paper was to simply test how effective chiropractic adjustments are for common migraines.

How They Did it

- This study was a randomized controlled trial period
- It lasted six months
- The trial included three stages which were two months of data prior to the treatment, Two months of data during treatment, and two months of data following treatment period
- The comparisons were made at the end of the six months for the chiropractic adjustment group as well as a control group.
- 127 subjects were used period
- Their ages where between 10 years old and 70 years old.
- The protocols put forth by the international headache society were used in the diagnosis of migraines.
- The subjects had to experience a minimum of one migraine per month to be accepted to the study.
- The subjects underwent two months of chiropractic manipulative therapy. Which consisted of 16 treatments.
- The subjects completed detailed diaries throughout treatment.

What They Found

- The treatment group shows significant improvement in frequency, duration, disability, and medication use.
- In other words, 22% had a greater than 90% reduction of migraines.

"The results of this study support previous results showing that some people report significant improvement in migraines after chiropractic spinal manipulative therapy. A high percentage (>80%) of participants reported stress as a major factor for their migraines. It appears probable that chiropractic care has an effect on the physical conditions related to stress and that in these people the effects of the migraine are reduced[84]."

DON'T HOLD BACK ON CHIROPRACTIC FOR YOUR HEADACHE

There is no doubt in my mind that the majority of headaches could be eliminated if the right treatment were to be used from the start. It may be anecdotal experience, but it is still personal, clinical experience nonetheless. Personal experience has shown me time and time again that chiropractic manipulation is highly effective in treating headaches.

Certainly specific types of headaches such as tension-type headaches and cervicogenic headaches, respond extremely well to chiropractic treatment.

In fact, my own "guesstimate" from over 19 years of experience is that about 80% of headaches respond very well, 10% get better but don't go completely away, and only 10% or so cannot be treated with chiropractic. Those are pretty solid odds if one is having debilitating headaches of just about any kind.

If someone said they could give me an 80% probability of something happening, I would likely bet a good amount of money on it.

Why They Did It

There are really two thought processes when it comes to conservative treatment of headaches. One is the chiropractic manipulation, also commonly called the "adjustment." Then there is the term in the traditional medical field called mobilization. With mobilization, they commonly add exercises to the treatment protocol.

There have been no studies directly comparing the two types of treatment to each other in terms of their effectiveness. The authors in this study wanted to test which was the better regimen for cervicogenic headaches specifically.

How They Did It

- 110 people suffering from cervicogenic headaches participated.
- The 110 participants were randomly placed into either a manipulation group or a mobilization group.
- The outcome or result was measured by the numeric Pain Rating Scale.
- Headache frequency, duration, and disability were measured as well using the Neck Disability Index, medication intake, and Global Rating of Change.
- Treatment lasted for 4 weeks and patients were assessed at a follow-up appointment 1 week after the end of treatment, 4 weeks after the end of treatment, and 3 months after the end of treatment.

What They Found

- Those in the Chiropractic Manipulation group showed significantly less intensity in their headache symptoms than did the other group that only had mobilization and exercise.
- The patients in the Chiropractic Manipulation group also had significantly less frequency of the headache symptoms.
- Not only did the outcomes show manipulation to be superior, but patients in the Chiropractic Manipulation group also felt greater improvement themselves based on self reports.

"Six to eight sessions of upper cervical and upper thoracic manipulation were shown to be more effective than mobilization and exercise in patients with chronic headache, and the effects were maintained at 3 months[81]."

CHIROPRACTIC VS. AMITRIPTYLINE FOR MIGRAINES GRUDGE MATCH

It has been my experience that most people identify chiropractors with being practitioners for back and neck pain, but not necessarily for headaches or migraines.

Research has shown that for many headaches and migraines, once an emergency is ruled out, doctors of chiropractic should be the entry point into the healthcare system.

Here's research for it.

Why They Did It
They estimate that around 11 million Americans have moderate to severe disability from migraines. The authors wanted to get a closer reading on how effective spinal manipulation is on migraine headaches.

How They Did It
- 218 Randomized patients pre-diagnosed with migraines
- Measure efficacy of spinal manipulation
- Measured efficacy of amitriptyline
- Measured efficacy of treatment that combines both manipulation AND amitriptyline

- Clinically important improvement observed with the patients undergoing spinal manipulation alone (40%)
- Improvement under amitriptyline (49%)
- Improvement in the group undergoing both treatments. (41%)
- BUT......upon post-treatment evaluation, A FAR HIGHER AMOUNT OF MIGRAINE PATIENTS THAT UNDERWENT SPINAL MANIPULATION ALONE HAD REDUCTION ON THEIR HEADACHE DISABILITY INDEX SCORES THAN IN THE OTHER TWO GROUPS.

Wrap It Up

Since the study proved that Chiropractic was equal in effectiveness to a an established medical treatment (amitriptyline), then Chiropractic should be considered the reasonable option in complaints such as these[36].

CHIROPRACTIC EFFECTIVE FOR HEADACHES AND MIGRAINES

I can't tell you how many patients come in to see chiropractors for headaches. I've seen them range from life-long headaches/migraines all the way to, "I woke up this morning with a headache."

I have had different levels of success with headaches too. My most memorable success was a patient that had them her entire life. She had nuclear bone scans. She had injections in the back of her head. She had MRI's that came back normal. Yet, she continued to be plagued by them daily.

After initializing treatment, it literally took only two weeks and she stopped having headaches right then and there. That was years ago and she still does not suffer from headaches!

I've had the headaches be a little "stubborn" too. One patient in the last year comes to mind. She was in her 50's and has been plagued with them since she was a child. We treated her with marginal success for about 3 weeks.

I'm a firm believer that if we're not getting results we either need to change what we're doing, or I'm not the guy for this patient. So we began including cold laser in her treatment.

Viola! That was it. She's doing great and still having no headaches.

We DO, from time to time, run into a headache that won't respond to treatment but that is a rare occasion and is probably only around 10%-15% of the headache patients. Chiropractic just works with headaches. Here's more proof!

Why They Did It:
Since chronic headaches have a substantial socioeconomic impact, the authors/researchers were interested in what part spinal manipulative therapy (SMT) could play in helping the situation.

How They Did It:
- Randomized clinical trials
- The trials had to include, at the least, one patient-related outcome measure
- They used a search of MEDLINE and EMBASE databases to find trials that fit the protocol
- They used all data from Cumulative Index of Nursing and Allied Health Literature
- They used the Chiropractic Research Archives Collection,
- They used the Manual, Alternative, and Natural Therapies Information System
- Nine trials involving 683 patients

What They Found

- Moderate evidence that SMT has significantly more effectiveness than massage in cervicogenic headaches.
- SMT has effect comparable to common prescription medications for tension and migraine headaches.

Wrap It Up

More studies need to be conducted over longer periods of time but, with these studies being randomized clinical trials, the evidence shows chiropractic to be very effective for headaches and migraines while avoiding medication and their associated side effects[30].

MANIPULATION & EXERCISE

WHY CHIROPRACTIC IS THE SECRET WEAPON FOR BACK & NECK PAIN

Why They Did It

As stated above, the authors felt there were a multitude of randomized clinical trials, reviews, and national clinical guidelines regarding chiropractic for low back and neck pain but that there still remained some controversy as to its effectiveness among some in the medical field. They wanted to step back and review all of the information, only accept valuable papers on the topic, and generate a solid opinion on chiropractic effectiveness for treating low back and neck pain.

How They Did It

- They chose papers on randomized trials from around the world through computerized databases.
- They used two independent reviewers to check the quality of the papers using guidelines laid out before starting the project.
- 69 randomized clinical trials were reviewed.
- Only 43 ultimately met the predetermined criteria and were accepted for the review.

What They Found

- There is moderate evidence that Chiropractic has more effectiveness for short-term pain relief than does mobilization and limited evidence of faster recovery over physical therapy.

- For chronic low back pain, there is moderate evidence showing that spinal manipulative therapy has an effect that is equal to prescription non-steroidal anti-inflammatory drug. Also, spinal manipulation and mobilization show effectiveness in short-term relief over that of a primary practitioner as well as superiority in the long term when compared to physical therapy.
- There is moderate to limited evidence showing that Chiropractic is superior to physical therapy in the long term and the short-term treatment of low back pain and neck pain.
- For a mix of short and long term pain, Chiropractic was either similar or superior to McKenzie exercises, medical treatment, or physical therapy.

Wrap It Up

The authors concluded that "recommendations can be made with confidence regarding the use of spinal manipulative therapy and/or mobilization as a viable option for the treatment of both low back pain and neck pain[33]."

YOU SHOULD KNOW THIS ABOUT OVERALL STIFFNESS

Why They Did It

Throughout the years, there have been several studies on spinal manipulative treatment. However, none have specifically addressed its effectiveness for stiffness. This particular paper aimed to evaluate spinal stiffness in patients having lower back pain and their results following spinal manipulative therapy.

How They Did It
- Patients with lower back pain had two adjustments in one week.
- Outcome assessment was based on the Oswestry Disability Index.
- They evaluated spinal stiffness using ultrasonic measures and mechanized indentation measures.
- The measurements were taken before and after each adjustment as well as a week following the last treatment.

What They Found
- There was a quick and significant decrease in stiffness overall as well as terminal stiffness.
- The decrease in stiffness was noted after the adjustment.
- The improvement of the outcome assessment testing was due to the significant decrease in stiffness.

Wrap It Up
The researchers found significant correlation with immediate and post-adjustment stiffness decrease and ultimate outcome assessment. The results seem to point to a relationship between changes in stiffness and outcomes through the use of spinal adjustments that aren't seen without the adjustment.

This study was supported by the National Institutes of Health[97].

CHRONIC NECK PAIN AND REHAB EXERCISE COMBINED

This paper spotlights the benefits of spinal manipulation in CHRONIC NECK PAIN - not only the benefits of spinal manipulation, but also the addition of rehab exercises as part of the treatment regimen.

WHY THEY DID IT

The authors wanted to contrast the effectiveness of spinal manipulation when combined with low-tech rehab, MedX rehab, or spinal manipulation alone over the course of 2 years. Of the research available, the authors did not feel that there was adequate research outside of short-term follow-ups.

HOW DID THEY DO IT?

- 191 patients with chronic neck pain
- Patients were randomized to 11 weeks in one of the three treatment protocols.
- The patients self-reported on questionnaires measuring pain, disability, general health status, improvement, satisfaction, and medication use.
- The questionnaires were collected after 5 and 11 weeks of treatment
- They were also collected after 3, 6, 12, and 24 months after treatment concluded

WHAT DID THEY FIND?

- 93% of the patients finished the 11 weeks of treatment.
- 76% provided the required information at all points of treatment and follow-up.
- There was a difference in the patient-rated pain in favor of the two exercise groups
- There was a difference in satisfaction with care when spinal manipulation was combined with rehab exercises.

WRAP It Up

There was a clear advantage of spinal manipulation combined with exercise vs. spinal manipulation alone over two years. The researchers concluded that chronic neck pain patients should enter treatment protocols including rehab exercises along with spinal manipulation for optimal results[63].

CHIROPRACTIC &
EXERCISE TOGETHER. MORE BENEFICIAL?

Why They Did It

It has been common knowledge for some time now that low-grade exercises and stretching can help one in the process of overcoming low back pain. Years ago, the recommendation was to go home, lie down, and get plenty of bed rest. That's not the case anymore.

There have been several studies that have shown how effective spinal manipulation, spinal mobilization, chiropractic adjustments are for low back pain for both ACUTE and CHRONIC conditions.

So, what would be the cumulative effect from the use of both in patients with low back pain?

How They Did It?

- This study was a randomized controlled trial.
- They were separated into groups: Manual Therapy group and Exercise group.
- They took 49 patients having chronic low back pain and/or pain into the leg.
- They were of the ages 20-60 years old
- They underwent 16 treatments over eight weeks
- Each treatment in the Manual Therapy group lasted approximately 45 minutes and consisted of manual adjustments as well as 11 exercises targeting flexibility, strength, and coordination
- Each treatment in the Exercise Therapy group lasted 45 minutes with a 35-minute focus on the torso, trunk, and legs followed by a 10-minute exercise bicycle cool-down
- Their progress was measured before treatment, immediately after treatment, at 4 weeks, 6 months, and at one year after treatment

What Did They Find?

- Both groups showed improvement
- The MANUAL-THERAPY GROUP had greater, more significant improvement over the Exercise Therapy group in ALL outcome assessment reports at ALL points in the follow-ups.
- Pain in the Manual Therapy group reduced DOUBLE that of the Exercise Therapy group.
- The Manual-Therapy group was 40% more likely to return to work after treatment than the Exercise Therapy group patients.
- At the one-year follow-up, there was only a 19% instance of the Manual Therapy group being sick-listed compared to 59% in the Exercise Therapy group.

Wrap Up

What a difference. This shows definitively that exercise is most certainly beneficial but in conjunction with manual therapy, it cannot be beat[98].

THE UK BEAM STUDY: CHIROPRACTIC & EXERCISE IS THE WAY TO GO FOR BACK PAIN

A wide spread study was carried out in the UK for their National Health Service (NHS). It concerned researching the effectiveness of exercise alone, manipulation/mobilization alone, and then the two combined for the treatment of back pain.

Why They Did It

The authors wanted to explore the effectiveness of the three options for treatment of back pain for possible recommendations in the National Health Service for the UK primary practitioners.

Jeff S. Williams, DC, FIANM

How They Did It
- This study was a pragmatic randomized trial.
- They used 181 general practices
- 63 community settings in 14 centers in the UK
- 1334 patients were used in the study.
- The Roland-Morris disability questionnaire was used for the Outcome Assessments at the 3-month mark and at the 12-month mark.

What They Found
- All groups improved somewhat over time.
- Exercise helped at the 3-month mark.
- Manipulation was effective at the 3-month mark as well as the 12-month mark.
- Manipulation followed by Exercise was even more effective at both marks.

Wrap It Up
When compared to "best care" practices for general practitioners in the UK's NHS system, Manipulation followed by Exercise was the moderately better overall treatment for back pain[20].

DISC BULGES, HERNIATIONS, RADICULOPATHY, NEUROPATHY

I want to preface the discussion on discs by talking about the MRI reports that come back from radiologists.

MRIs are traditionally performed in the supine (lying on the back) position. This position removes any weight-bearing (axial loading) or gravity from the equation of forces acting on the disc.

I have never experienced a radiologist stating in a report that the disc is herniated 3 mm posteriorly but that upon sitting or weight-bearing, it will likely increase the posterior displacement to 5mm or more. I do not fault the radiologists on this. It is not their job to guess but rather to be objective and report what is on the image.

I have had a handful of discussions with radiologists, In our discussions, I have asked them if a herniation will increase upon weight-bearing. It has always made sense to me that gravity and pressure from weight-bearing would indeed cause the size of the herniation to increase. However, they ALL felt that the disc was too strong for that to be the case.

Luckily, I am not the only practitioner that had this question in mind. It has actually been researched and, through research, we can demonstrate that the disc does indeed increase in size upon weight-bearing.

Thanks to the research done on this topic, we can communicate more effectively with our patients concerning their MRI results.

CAN DISC HERNIATIONS ACTUALLY BE WORSE THAN THE MRI SHOWS? – PART I

A question I have asked myself over the years is, "Yes, this patient has a low back disc herniation of 4 mm (or whatever it may be) when laying down in a tube doing an MRI but...what happens to that disc when a person sits up or bends over? What happens to it while bearing weight?"

This is a valid question when you consider that I have seen patients with classic disc signs including radiculopathy into one or more feet. Understand that a general rule with radiculopathy, according to Dr. Donald Murphy's CRISP Protocol book, is that the further beyond the knee it extends, the more likely it is to be a disc causing the symptom. In these patients, when you have several other orthopedic signs pointing to a disc, you would reasonably expect a mild to moderate, or possibly a severe, disc herniation.

Per the thinking of Robin McKenzie, DPT, the disc can migrate and be likened to a really strong bag of water. If I lean one direction, I will push the bulk of the material in the opposite direction and vice versa.

Also consider that the most pressure you can put on your lower back is to be in the seated position or seated and bending forward position. Even more so when load is added to the mix. What exactly do these positions and loads do to a disc that is already at 4 mm when lying down without bearing any weight?

What do we do when we have questions? We turn to research and thank goodness I'm not the only one that felt this was an important question to figure out!

As a matter of fact, I found a good number of research papers on this topic. So many that I am going to break the discussion (and sections) into separate parts to make it easier to digest.

We'll start Part I with a study by Nguyen et. al. called "Upright magnetic resonance imaging of the lumbar spine: Back and Pain Radiculopathy."

Why They Did It
While low back pain and pain into the legs or numbness and tingling into the legs may be somewhat common, many times the findings on an MRI don't show what we would expect to see. The authors of this study wanted to find out what difference there would be in a supine, (lying down) MRI vs. an MRI performed with the patient in a seated position bearing weight (axial loaded).

How They Did It
- There were a total of 17 participants.
- 10 of the participants were asymptomatic.
- Seven of the participants were symptomatic.
- Upright MRI was done on each adult while they were in the seated position.
- Measurements were performed from the second and third lumbar level (beginning of the low back) down to the fifth lumbar and tailbone region.
- There were also measurements of the areas the nerves of the low back pass through to determine the various sizes of these holes, also known as foramen.

What They Found
- Mid-disc width accounted for 56% of the maximum foramen with in the symptomatic group.
- Mid-disc width was over 63% of the maximum foramen within asymptomatic volunteers.
- Disc bulging was 48% larger in the symptomatic group.
- The measurements of the foramen were smaller in the symptomatic group.

Wrap It Up

The information suggests that MRIs performed in the upright, seated position can be useful in the diagnosis process because it is better able to distinguish important differences among the asymptomatic and symptomatic. Especially in regards to the size of the intervertebral foramen[99].

In another study by Madsen, et. al., while the authors argue that axial loading of the spine does not necessarily cause any significant changes to the disc itself, the simple act of having more extension in the spine was a determining factor as to how much space remained in the dural sac surrounding the spinal cord or cauda equina[100].

I wanted to be fair so I included this study. It suggests the discs play a very small part in the process but, as you will see from approximately 10 other papers we will discuss, this sort of finding or thought process is very much in the minority.

In yet another similar study (Hansson, et. al.) the authors were testing similar parameters in the cases of diagnosed stenosis patients.

Why They Did It

Protrusion of a disc has commonly been cited as the cause of symptoms from nerve root compression in patients with stenosis when the spine was axially loaded (weight-bearing). They were interested in determining whether it is the disc or the ligamentum flavum that caused the difference when loaded.

How They Did It
- There were 24 participants in the study.
- The lumbar (low back) spines were examined by MRI while lying down supine (face up).
- Then the study was repeated with roughly half of their weight loaded to the spine axially.

- The measurements were through the cross-sectional areas of the spinal canal as well as the ligamentum flavum, the thickness of the ligamentum flavum, the posterior bulge of the disc and the intervertebral angle.

What They Found
- The axial loading did in fact decrease the cross-sectional size of the spinal canal.
- Increased bulge or thickening of the ligamentum flavum was to blame for 50%-85% of the decrease in the spinal canal size.

Wrap It Up
The authors concluded that it appears the ligamentum flavum, not the disc, played a dominate role in reducing the size of the spinal canal on axially loaded spines for those with stenosis[101].

CAN DISC HERNIATIONS ACTUALLY BE WORSE THAN THE MRI SHOWS? – PART II

My question, as stated in Part I of this series, was, "If a low back (or lumbar) disc is 4 mm herniated while laying down in an MRI tube, what happens when the patient then sits up and becomes weight-bearing? Will the herniation increase or be affected at all?"

Continuing with Part II of this discussion, we'll start with this study by DS Choy, et. al. called "Magnetic resonance imaging of the lumbosacral spine under compression.

Why They Did It
1. Evidently sitting MRI imaging exists at Harvard and Zurich. Since most MRI machines can't accomplish this sort of imaging, the author of the paper wanted to see if, in a regular machine, compression could be dependably added to the spine in order to duplicate the pressures found in the low back discs while people are in the seated position.

How They Did It

The author created a plywood compression frame able to be used in a standard MRI machine. When applied, the patient lying in the MRI machine would be subject to similar compression forces as those experienced when seated.

What They Found

They could reproduce the symptoms in 50% of the patients through the compression. Here's the finding that led me to include this study in this discussion: the author was able to also reproduce "augmentation" or accentuate the disc herniation from applying the compression.

Wrap It Up

The compression applied allowed the author to reproduce the forces experienced when a person sits, it reproduced the symptomatology in half of the subjects, and the compression caused the disc to herniate further[102].

Continuing with the second paper: it's by Nowicki, et. al. called, "Occult lumbar lateral spinal stenosis in neural foramina subjected to physiologic loading," from 1996.

Why They Did It

These authors were interested in how different positioning of the trunk affects the relationships of the bones and discs in regards to the neural structures in the same anatomic region. They also wanted to find out how disc degeneration responds to loading.

How They Did It

- The authors used cadavers for this study and looked at each vertebral segment (L1 on L2 or S1 on L5 for example) via CT or MRI scans.
- The study was done "loaded, frozen in situ, reexamined with CT, and sectioned with a cryomicrotome."

- The neural foramina (holes the spinal nerves run through) were classified as follows
  . No evident stenosis
  . Having stenosis
  . Having occult stenosis
  . Showing resolved stenosis
- Also studied was "the effect of spinal level, disc type, and load type on the prevalence of stenosis."

What They Found

The average finding in the paper were that extension, flexion, lateral bending, and rotation show contact or compression of the spinal nerve by the ligamentum flavum or disc in 18% of the neural foramina. Extension loading produced the most cases of nerve root contact. Disc degeneration significantly increased the prevalence of pain stenosis.

Wrap It Up

The authors concluded, "The study supports the concept of dynamic spinal stenosis; that is, intermittent stenosis of the neural foramina. Flexion, extension, lateral bending, and axial rotation significantly changed the anatomic relationships of the ligamentum flavum and intervertebral disc to the spinal nerve roots[103]."

We are starting to understand that positioning and weight-bearing does indeed have an affect on the discs, the ligamentum flavum, and the neural structures present at each level.

Here's the last one we will cover in Part II called "The diagnostic effect from axial loading of the lumbar spine during computed tomography and magnetic resonance imaging in patients with degenerative disorders." It was published in the prestigious Spine journal.

Why They Did It

While imaging through CT or MRI scans is becoming more popular these days, they are still performed in the supine, or unloaded, position. Basically, people are lying down in a tube rather than sitting or standing, thus, bearing weight.

The authors stated goal in this paper were to find out if there was any real value in imaging patients that had axial loads (simulated weight-bearing) applied in cases of degenerative spines.

How They Did It
- Device was used to induce a load on the low back before imaging.
- 172 patients were examined with compression applied.
- 50 of those were imaged with CTs.
- 122 of those subjects were imaged with MRIs.
- Any change in the major anatomy of the regions was noted.

What They Found

"Additional valuable information was found" in 50 of the original 172 participants. "A narrowing of the lateral recess causing compression of the nerve root was found at 42 levels in 35 patients at axial loading."

Wrap It Up

There is certainly and frequently additional information that can be gathered for diagnostic purposes when the imaging is done with weigh-bearing loads applied. This included those with neurogenic claudication as a result of stenosis but also sciatica[104].

Jeff S. Williams, DC, FIANM

CAN DISC HERNIATIONS ACTUALLY BE WORSE THAN THE MRI SHOWS? – PART III

Welcome to Part III of the series we have been doing called, "Can Disc Herniations Actually Be Worse Than The MRI Shows?"

My question, as stated in Part I and Part II of this series, is, "If a low back (or lumbar) disc is 4 mm herniated while laying down in an MRI tube, what happens when the patient then sits up and becomes weight-bearing? Will the herniation increase or be affected at all?"

Let's start Part III with a paper called, "Evaluation of intervertebral disc herniation and hypermobile intersegmental instability in symptomatic adult patients undergoing recumbent and upright MRI of the cervical or lumbosacral spines." by Ferreiro Perez, et al.

Why They Did It
The authors had the same question in mind when they went about this study. They wanted to simply figure out the difference between MRIs done lying down and those done when in the seated position.

How They Did It
- 89 Patients studied
- 45 of them had their low back imaged
- 44 patients had their necks imaged
- The images were done in both the lying down position as well as the sitting.

What They Found
- The overall combined recumbent (lying down) miss rate in cases of pathology was 15%
- Overall combined recumbent underestimation rate in cases of pathology was 62%
- Overall combined upright-seated underestimation in cases of pathology was 16%.

Wrap It Up

Upright-seated MRIs were seen to be superior to recumbent MRIs in 52 of the patients studied for conditions of posterior disc herniation and spondylolisthesis. Recumbent MRIs were only superior in 12% of the patients[105].

The second paper we'll cover is called "Effect of intervertebral disk degeneration on spinal stenosis during magnetic resonance imaging with axial loading" by Ahn et al.

Why They Did It

They wanted to determine if disc degeneration will increase the severity of spinal stenosis when the spine is loaded with axial pressure.

How They Did It

- 51 patients having symptoms of neurogenic intermittent claudication and/or sciatica had MRI imaging loaded as well as non-loaded.
- All foramen and the spinal canal that neurologic structures run through were measured for changes in size.

What They Found

"More accurate diagnosis of stenosis can be achieved using MR imaging with axial loading, especially if grade 2 to 4 disk degeneration is present."

Wrap It Up

Seated or loaded MRIs are superior for diagnostic purposes[106].

The last study we'll look at in this section is called "Dynamic effects on the lumbar spinal canal: axially loaded CT-myelography and MRI in patients with sciatica and/or neurogenic claudication" by Willen et al.

Why They Did It
The authors did this one for the same reason as the others; to find out if seated MRIs can give us more accurate diagnostic information in regard to those suffering neurologic symptoms resulting from disc herniations.

How They Did It
- 50 subjects imaged with CT
- 34 were imaged through MRI
- The imaging was performed lying down as well as with an axial load applied.
- Measurements of the anatomy were made to be able to distinguish any differences the loading may bring about.

What They Found
"Axial loading of the lumbar spine in computed tomographic scanning and magnetic resonance imaging is recommended in patients with sciatica or neurogenic claudication when the dural sac cross-sectional area at any disc location is below 130 mm2 in conventional psoas-relaxed position and when there is a suspected narrowing of the dural sac or the nerve roots, especially in the ventrolateral part of the spinal canal in psoas-relaxed position"

Wrap It Up
The value of the diagnostic information is significantly greater when the subject has an axial load applied during the imaging process[107].

CAN DISC HERNIATIONS ACTUALLY BE WORSE THAN THE MRI SHOWS? – PART IV

My question, as stated in Parts I, II, and III of this series, is, "If a low back (or lumbar) disc is 4 mm herniated while laying down in an MRI tube, what happens when the patient then sits up and becomes weight-bearing? Will the herniation increase or be affected at all?"

I'm hoping you've found this interesting and it can help you decipher the information on your MRIs better going forward.

Let's start Part IV with a paper called, "Axial loading during magnetic resonance imaging in patients with lumbar spinal canal stenosis: does it reproduce the positional change of the dural sac detected by upright myelography?" by Kanno et. al.

Why They Did It
The objective was to answer the same question. Does an axial loaded MRI change the anatomy of the vertebral segments including the neural structures?

How They Did It
- 44 patients participated.
- Imaging was done in the conventional manner and in the axial loaded manner.
- The size of the dural sack (the sack around the spinal cord) was measured in each type of imaging.

What They Found
- The size of the dural sack was significantly reduced in the axial loaded imaging.
- "The axial loaded MRI detected severe constriction with a higher sensitivity (96.4%) and specificity (98.2%) than the conventional MRI."

Wrap It Up
MRIs performed with axial loads showed significant changes in the size of the dural sack diameters. The axial loaded MRI is useful in representing positional changes similar to those experienced when upright and weight-bearing[108].

Next, we cover a paper called, "Axially loaded magnetic resonance image of the lumbar spine in asymptomatic individuals." This paper was done by Danielson et. al. in 2001.

Why They Did It

"To evaluate the effect of axial loading on asymptomatic individuals, as compared with the effect on patients who have clinical signs of lumbar spinal canal stenosis, and to assess the effect that different magnitude and duration of the applied load have on the dural cross-sectional area."

How They Did It

- MRIs were performed lying down as well as upright on the participants.
- The axial loading was performed lying down, face up with a "compression device" made for this study specifically.
- Degenerative changes were noted in and around the spinal canal.
- The diameter of the dural sack was measure in the lying down and in the upright position.

What They Found

The authors said, "A significant decrease in dural cross-sectional area from psoas-relaxed position to axial compression in extension was found in 24 individuals (56%), most frequently at L4-L5, and increasingly with age."

Wrap It Up

Using axial loaded MRI imaging demonstrated a significant reduction in the size of the dural sack, definitely in the patients already suffering symptoms.

There you have it. Since beginning this series, we have covered 12 research papers dealing with this topic specifically and it is exceedingly clear that indeed, upright or axial loaded MRIs are significantly superior to MRIs performed in the lying down position in regard to diagnosing herniated disc severity.

If your MRI says 4 mm and was performed in the lying down position, then it is a researched reality that the actual size of the disc herniation will likely be variable and much more significant with weight bearing activities. These include bending to the side, bending forward, bending backward, and performing activities of daily living and work responsibilities[109].

TESTED AND PROVEN: CAN YOU AVOID DISC HERNIATION SURGERY?

Why They Did It

There was a noted vacuum in the research literature in regards how a low back disc herniation progresses, regress, or simply exists through time. Nor were there any clear protocols or indications for when operations should be performed on low back disc herniations. In addition, there were clear indications in the literature suggesting that the largest of disc herniations showed the most likelihood of resolving. The paper wanted to explore whether the larger herniations are able to be treated through conservative management successfully.

How They Did It

- MRI imaging and Clinical Assessment were used.
- Clinical Assessment included the Lasegue test and a neurological exam.
- 37 patients met the criteria to be included in the study.
- The assessments and imaging were utilized over a 2-year period.
- The Oswestry Disability Index (ODI) questionnaire was used to assess function.

- The first follow-up appointment averaged 23.2 months out from the beginning of the study.
- At the first follow-up, 83% of the patients had COMPLETE and SUSTAINED recovery.
- The ODI went from 58% disability to 15% disability.
- The MRI imaging showed average reduction of the disc herniation by 64%!

Wrap It Up

"A massive disc herniation can pursue a favorable clinical course. If early progress is shown, the long-term prognosis is very good and even massive disc herniations can be treated conservatively[110]."

CHIROPRACTIC ADJUSTMENTS FOR LUMBAR DISC HERNIATIONS?

Why They Did It

They performed the study to estimate the effectiveness of chiropractic adjustments in patients that had lumbar disc herniations that were confirmed through the use of MRI imaging. They wanted to see if there was a difference between those conditions that were acute and chronic.

How They Did It

- It was a prospective cohort study.
- 148 patients included.
- Patients were between 18 and 65
- All had low back pain
- All had leg pain
- All had lumbar herniations that were confirmed through MRI imaging
- Outcomes were through self-assessed questionnaires at different time periods

What They Found

- There was significant improvement on all out come assessment questionnaires for all time intervals.
- 3 months post-treatment, 90.5% of patients were "improved"
- 1 year post-treatment, 88% were "improved"
- "Although acute patients improved faster by 3 months, 81.8% of chronic patients reported "improvement" with 89.2% "improved" at 1 year. There were no adverse events reported."

Wrap It Up

"A large percentage of acute and importantly chronic lumbar disc herniation patients treated with chiropractic spinal manipulation reported clinically relevant improvement[57]."

HOW RESEARCH MAY CHANGE HOW WE ALL VIEW LOW BACK DISC TREATMENT

Why They Did It

The authors in this paper were curious as to the safety and effectiveness of mobilization/manipulation of a lumbar disc herniation.

How They Did It

- The authors extracted the pertinent information from commonly used research databases such as PubMed, OVID, Cochrane Library, CBM, CNKI, and VIP.
- 832 papers on the topic (lumbar disc herniations) were extracted for the study.
- 8 of the papers actually met the criteria for the study and were subsequently used.
- There were 911 low back disc herniation patients within the qualifying 8 articles.
- The data was processed using the Cochrane systematic review process.

What They Found
The cure rate for those undergoing chiropractic manipulative treatments was greater than with other treatment methods, which included acupuncture, traction, thermotherapy, etc.

Wrap It Up
"This study shows that manipulative treatment on lumbar disc herniation is safe, effective, and both cure rate and the effective rate is better than other therapies." However, the authors also admit that higher quality evidence needs to be collected for a higher level of validation[31].

CAN CHIROPRACTIC EASE A HERNIATED CERVICAL DISC?

Why They Did It
Disc herniations in the neck is the second most common reason to have radiating symptoms from the neck region.

Swiss researchers decided to get some research done on the condition by attempting to assess the efficacy of spinal manipulative therapy in cervical disc complaints.

How They Did It
- 50 patients having neck disc issues confirmed via MRI
- The patients were aged 18-65.
- They all had pain in common neurological patterns (dermatomes).
- They also had sensory and/or motor changes corresponding to the nerve root indicated.
- At minimum, one positive orthopedic test for radiculopathy was required in order to be accepted into the study.
- They were treated with chiropractic adjustments three times per week.

- The Numeric Rating System (NRS) was used in the Outcome Assessment measures.
- The Neck Disability Index (NDI) was used in the Outcome Assessment measure. The subjects were assessed at 2 weeks, 4 weeks, and at the three-month marks.

What They Found
- Two weeks later over 55.3% of the patients improved significantly
- At 3 months, 85.7% had significant result
- None of them had any negative affects.

Wrap It Up
"Spinal manipulative therapy (chiropractic adjustments) for acute, subacute, and chronic patients with cervical disc herniations in this study produced significant improvement in symptoms with no adverse effects[111]."

Jeff S. Williams, DC, FIANM

NON-SURGICAL SPINAL DECOMPRESSION

After discussing MRI results in the low back, discussing the poor effectiveness for epidural spinal injections, discussing poor surgical outcomes, the goal of this section is to demonstrate effective protocols for treating disc complaints.

Let me be clear; non-surgical spinal decompression, according to all insurance plans to my knowledge, is still considered 'experimental and investigational'. In addition, you will likely find many practitioners in favor of using the modality and many that prefer to wait until there is more research available showing effectiveness.

Personally, I can only offer anecdotal evidence and experience from years of utilizing the modality and all of it is positive. Still, recalling the research pyramid, anecdotal evidence means little.

At the end of the day, I would most certainly like to see more research validating and proving the results I have seen over the years anecdotally.

When we discuss lack of effectiveness for a safe, non-invasive, non-pharmacological treatment modality, we should always remember something in the back of our minds; what treatment is the alternative? Even if there is a feeling of a lack of evidence for effectiveness but the modality is harmless and the alternative is injections, pain medication, and/or surgery, then what exactly is the harm in performing a test trial of treatment to assess for effectiveness and improvement?

Are we not charged with 'first, do no harm'?

With that acknowledgement, I provide the following for consideration:

IMPRESSIVE EFFECTIVENESS SHOWN IN SPINAL DECOMPRESSION MEDICAL STUDY

In disc complaints and facet arthropathy, spinal decompression should literally be the entry point into the healthcare system and surgery should be the exit point from the healthcare system. The evidence shows it to be true.

In recent research, injections for these conditions offers little to zero effectiveness and the risks outweigh any perceived reward. Physical therapy is minimally effective in disc conditions. Even chiropractic adjustments are limited in disc complaints.

Surgery can be effective but at what cost? Also, many disc conditions simply heal after some period of time.

A good argument can be made for chiropractic and non-surgical spinal decompression being an answer to faster, more conservative pain relief in disc complaints.

Why They Did It

Since herniated and degenerated discs have been shown to have elevated pressures within them that are then elevated further through standing and sitting, the question is, "Can the disc be decompressed, thus allowing proper healing and repair of the herniation and annular tears while rehydrating the disc at the same time?"

The goal was to answer that question in an objective and quantifiable manner.

How They Did It
- They took Pre- and Post- treatment MRIs.
- 18 patients: 12 males, 8 females. Ages 26-74.
- Pain or numbness (due to herniated discs) into the lower limbs was present in 14 of the patients.
- Pain or numbness (due to facet arthropathy and stenosis) was present in 6 patients.
- 20 Decompression treatments were given in 4-5 weeks
- 2 patients received 40 treatments over 8 weeks.
- Decompression was performed at 1/2 of the patient's body weight plus 10 lbs.
- Clinical status assessed before, during, and after along with the standard analog pain rating scale and a neurological exam as well just to be sure.

What They Found

MRI OUTCOMES
- Disc Herniation
  - 10 out of 14 patients improved SIGNIFICANTLY, some globally.
  - There were measured improvements in disc herniations
    - 0% in 2 of the patients
    - 20% in 4 of the patients
    - 30%-50% in 4 patients
    - 90% in 2 patients, which was the set of patients that received 40 treatments over 8 weeks.
- Facet Joint Arthropathy
  - No demonstrable change on the MRI alone except for 2 patients.

CLINICAL OUTCOMES
- Besides the MRI results, all except for 3 of the patients had VERY SIGNIFICANT pain relief.
- Besides the MRI results, all except for 3 of the patients had COMPLETE relief of weakness when present.

- Besides the MRI results, all except for 3 of the patients had COMPLETE relief of immobility and numbness.
- In disc herniation, 10 out of 14 experienced 10%-90% improvement in symptoms.

Wrap It Up

(Copied and Pasted from original article for accuracy)
- Decompression treatments afforded good or excellent relief of pain and disability whether from herniated disc or foraminal or lateral spinal stenosis.
- MRI showed imperfect correlation with degree of clinical improvement but 10% to 90% reduction in disc herniation size could be seen at least at the critical point of nerve root impingement in 10 of 14 patients.
- Two patients with extended courses of treatment showed 90% disc reduction and one of these had early rehydration of the degenerated disc at L4-5. An "empty pouch" sign on MRI at the site of previous herniation was seen in these 2 patients.
- Foraminal and lateral spinal or facet arthrosis cases causing radiculopathy without herniation also improved but without MRI change.
- Annulus healing or patching in the herniated disc can be shown by MRI and is postulated to be a primary factor in clinical and MRI improvement[112].

WHAT EVERYONE SHOULD KNOW ABOUT DISC HERNIATIONS & NON-SURGICAL SPINAL DECOMPRESSION

This week's research abstract has to do with the restoration of the height of the disc following decompression treatment.

Why They Did It

They wanted to find out if changes in low back pain due to disc degeneration would correlate with changes in lumbar disc height as measured by CT scans.

How They Did It

- They identified patients with chronic low back pain due to disc herniation
- They underwent a 6 week decompression treatment protocol
- The disc height was measured before treatment and after treatment via CT scans
- They measured pain on a verbal rating, 0-10.

What They Found

- During treatment, low back pain in the test subjects decreased from 6.2 to 1.6
- Disc height increased from 7.5mm to 8.8mm.

Wrap It Up

Spinal Decompression effectively and significantly reduced pain and increased disc height in the test subjects[113].

NON-SURGICAL SPINAL DECOMPRESSION: ENTRY POINT INTO THE SYSTEM FOR HERNIATED DISCS?

Should spinal decompression be the entry point into the healthcare system for herniated discs? Although my experience with spinal decompression in my practice is considered anecdotal, my opinion is "Absolutely. YES!"

I can tell you lots of great patients that we have had come through out doors that have avoided surgery and are back to normal lives as a result of spinal decompression.

But, luckily, one doesn't have to just take my word for it. There is actually research that shows how effective spinal decompression is.

Decompression has shown to be effective in re-hydrating the spinal discs, reducing the disc bulge itself, and decreasing pain over all. Not to mention the fact that we have had patients canceling their spinal surgeries for years now. I would say that is a pretty big deal!

Why They Did It

Since pain in the lumbosacral spine is the most common musculoskeletal pain and causes days out of work and it is the biggest cause of disability in people younger than 45 years of age, the authors wished to explore further whether or not spinal decompression could be an effective answer.

How They Did It

- The study was a randomized, Blinded study.
- Some patients were assigned to simple traction treatment.
- Some patients were assigned to decompression treatment
- Both the traction and decompression patients received weighted pools of 50% of their body weight +10 pounds.

What They Found

- 86% of ruptured intervertebral disc patients had improvement with spinal decompression
- There was significant relief from sciatica and back pain. In contrast, there were only 55% that had good improvement in the use of traction
- None of the traction patients achieved excellent results.
- In patients that had facet arthrosis 75% of them had good to excellent results with decompression.
- In the traction group, only 50% of the patients achieved good to excellent results.

Jeff S. Williams, DC, FIANM

Non-surgical spinal decompression was significantly more effective for disc herniation as well as facet arthrosis than was simple traction treatment. And it was certainly more effective than no treatment at all[114].

CAN SPINAL TRACTION HELP REHYDRATE A DEGENERATED DISC?

Non-surgical spinal decompression has shown phenomenal efficacy in our practice but there seems to be a relationship in patients' minds regarding insurance coverage and validity of the treatment.

In other words, many times our patients seem to initially think that if the insurance company doesn't cover a service (spinal decompression or cold laser) that it is probably of no use.

Of course, this is not true. If you were an insurance company and you had to pay out on all of the services doctors perform, would you be in any hurry to add more new services to your tab? Insurance companies are in the business of making money. They are not interested in figuring out ways they can spend more of it.

My way of educating patients is to demonstrate the proof. These research abstracts that I share aren't mostly performed and authored by chiropractors. These are government agencies, medical doctors, hospitals, colleges, PhDs, etc. If you cannot believe the validity of these people's findings, then you need to ask yourself, who CAN you believe then?

Here is one such research abstract I found for you.

Why They Did It

The goal here was to figure out the effect of traction (decompression) on the outer ring of the disc. Since decompression is conservative, certainly vs. surgery, it's a good thing to know its effectiveness in treating the disc.

The normal accepted benefits of traction/decompression have been an increase in the disc height, enlargement of the areas the spinal nerve roots pass through, and a decrease in the internal pressure of the disc itself. These are the benefits but they've not been investigated through research as thoroughly as they could be.

How They Did It

This excerpt is copied and pasted directly from the original abstract. Due to its specificity, I felt it important in the interest of accuracy:

- 48 thoracic discs were dissected from 8 porcine spines (140 kg, 6-month old) within 4 hours after killing them.
- They were divided into 3 groups: intact, degraded without traction, and degraded with traction.
- Each disc was incubated in a whole-organ culture system and subjected to diurnal loadings for 7 days.
- Except for the intact group, discs were degraded with 0.5 mL of trypsin on day 1 and a 5-hour fatigue loading on day 2. From day 4 to day 6, half of the degraded discs received a 30-minute traction treatment per day (traction force: 20 kg; loading: unloading = 30 s: 10 s). By the end of the incubation, the discs were inspected for disc height loss, annulus microstructure, molecular (fluorescein sodium) intensity, and cell viability.

What They Found

Transfer of molecules into and out of the disc decreased after degradation/degeneration of the disc. With traction treatment, however, the pores in the outer ring of the disc were opened up allowing for increased transfer of molecules, therefore allowing increased rehydration of the degenerated disc. This activity was not increased to the level of a fresh, brand new disc, but certainly increased from its previous condition.

The authors of the abstract concluded, "Traction treatment is effective in enhancing nutrition supply and promoting disc cell proliferation of the degraded discs[115]."

WHY GET SPINAL INJECTIONS WHEN CHIROPRACTIC IS AVAILABLE?

Continuing our theme of chiropractic reducing healthcare costs, being non-invasive and conservative, and being equally effective.... research in 2013 showed that **chiropractic adjustments were equally effective as epidural injections for those suffering from low back pain.** And that is minus the risk and without the significant costs that go along with the injections!

It concluded that conservative chiropractic care can significantly reduce pain seen in herniations of the lower back discs. Of course, it's less expensive too.

Side effects of steroids being injected into you are:
- Weakening of muscles in the area
- Weakening of the bone in the area
- Disruption of the body's natural hormone balance
- Lightening of your wallet

Although spinal injections are commonly prescribed, there is still a lot of controversy as to their effectiveness, especially when compared to other options that are safer and less invasive.

To my knowledge, there are 4 main treatment options for disc herniations:

1. Injections – they treat the inflammation, not the disc, and are usually short-lived and minimally effective.
2. Physical therapy – does not treat the disc specifically but can help with core strengthening
3. Surgery – certainly an effective option but a study I read recently stated that only about 30% are successful the first time.
4. Chiropractic Care With Spinal Decompression – I'm biased but this is the treatment of choice in a disc herniation in my opinion. It's safe, conservative, much more cost effective, and is outstandingly effective. Spinal decompression is a "game-changer" for disc conditions.

This new study comes to us from the Journal of Manual and Physiological Therapeutics in where Swiss researchers compared chiropractic spinal manipulative therapy (SMT) and epidural nerve root injections (NRI).

How They Did It
- There were 102 patients with symptomatic lumbar herniations that were confirmed via MRI.
- Following one month of treatment, the two groups had significant improvement.

What They Found
- 76.5% said they were "much better" or "better"
- 60% had a significant reduction in pain
- Injection patients:
- 62.7% said they were "much better" or "better"
- 53% had a significant reduction in pain
- None of the chiropractic patients went on to receive surgery, while 3 of the injection patients eventually underwent a surgical procedure.

Jeff S. Williams, DC, FIANM

Although chiropractic won, the outcomes were fairly close to the same. The next step was to compare the costs of the treatments. They could only take averages and the averages for one month of each treatment were as follows:

- Chiropractic care = $558.00
- Injections = $729.00 (this price did not include the associated costs such as clinicians, more than one injection, MRI, etc.)

Wrap It Up

All of this tells us that patients can get relief through Chiropractic rather than having to worry about the side effects of injections and steroids and they can do at a much lower price[28]!

Jeff S. Williams, DC, FIANM

LOW-LEVEL LASER (AKA COLD LASER)

6 FACTS ABOUT COLD LASER YOU SHOULD KNOW BEFORE THE NEXT INJURY

As the years go by, Cold Laser therapy gains more and more supportive research. Its effectiveness at this point really is not in question as low-level laser has made it into the recommendations from the American College of Physicians for first-line therapies for back pain[116].

Basically, the laser is used to emit a high intensity light that can treat chronic and acute pain while also stimulating healing and reducing inflammation (a common cause of pain).

1. Although it sounds like cutting edge technology, Cold Laser therapy has been around since the mid-1950s. The best part about cold laser is that it is non-invasive and produces virtually no heat. There are really very few side effects and only a handful of reasons that you would not use cold laser therapy.

2. The next thing you need to know about Cold Laser therapy is that it is not cold. It is a misnomer. It gained the name to signify the fact that it is not a cutting or burning laser. Some cold lasers can be detected with slight heat during the treatment but certainly nothing hot or cold.

3. Surgeons have begun using cold laser for post-operative incision healing to speed the healing and to reduce the scarring. Podiatrists are using cold laser for plantar fasciitis. We chiropractors use it extensively for muscle strains, ligament sprains, plantar fasciitis, inflammation, nerve pain, and to increase the speed of healing of soft tissues and musculoskeletal complaints.

4. A great aspect of cold laser therapy is that chronic conditions can be controlled through regular, periodic treatments, while acute conditions almost always fade rapidly. Cold Laser is not only excellent at reducing treatment time but it is cost-effective as well.
5. Some common results of cold laser therapy:
   - Rapid disappearance of pain
   - Strong reduction of inflammation
   - Rapid recovery from injury
   - Immediate improvement of blood circulation at the treatment site
   - Faster healing of virtually all soft tissue injury

Let's get to the research papers. This first paper we will discuss is from 2014.

Why They Did It
The authors were trying to evaluate the various effects of cold laser therapy on the dorsal root ganglia that had undergone chronic compression. Chronic compression of the dorsal root ganglia is seen commonly following physical injury of that intervertebral foramen causing nerve damage.

How They Did It
- The study was performed on rats
- The rats had artificial compression of the dorsal root ganglia in the fourth and fifth lumbar vertebrae to simulate chronic compression.
- Cold laser therapy was applied to test its effectiveness.

What They Found
Outcome assessments showed that cold laser significantly lessened the pain period.

Wrap It Up

Cold laser showed the ability to enhance neural regeneration following chronic compression of the dorsal root ganglia, which improved movement in the rats. In regards to the therapeutic effects of cold laser, there was reduction of inflammation[117].

This next paper has to do with cold laser's affect on chronic osteoarthritis in the knee.

Why They Did It

The authors of this paper we're looking to estimate what effect cold laser therapy would have in regard to pain and performance with patients suffering from chronic osteoarthritis of the knee.

How They Did It

- The study included 40 patients with osteoarthritis of the knee.
- They were randomly selected into different groups
- One group was a laser group
- The other was a placebo group
- Eight different points were treated in each session
- Cold laser was used two times each week for a month.
- They measured pain intensity upon resting and upon movement
- They measured knee function
- They measured walking statistics like duration and difficulty
- All measurements were taken before treatment and after treatment.

What they found

- The laser group showed significant reduction in pain intensity upon resting and upon movement.
- The laser group had a significant increase in function of the knee.

- The laser group showed significant increase and the ability to walk longer distance and longer periods when compared to the placebo group.

Wrap It Up

Cold laser was shown to be a significantly effective modality for pain relief and function in patients suffering from chronic osteoarthritis of the knee joint[118].

HOW EFFECTIVE IS COLD LASER FOR SWELLING AND PAIN?

Why They Did It

The purpose of this paper was to find out if cold laser could be an effective alternative in treating swelling and pain. Specifically, in this research abstract, they wished to answer the question following orthognathic surgery. Also known as jaw surgery.

How They Did It
- They took 10 healthy patients that had undergone the surgery in with similar procedures performed.
- They used cold laser inside the mouth as well as outside the mouth on one side.
- Application to the other side of the jaw was simulated. It was the placebo side.
- They then compared the two sides in regards to swelling and pain assessments.

What They Found
- At the immediate post-op assessment, there was no difference.
- Swelling decreased significantly on the treatment side on assessments at 3, 7, 15, and 30 days after the surgery.
- The patients also reported less intense pain on the treatment side at 24 hours and 3 days after surgery.

Jeff S. Williams, DC, FIANM

Through research, cold laser was shown to be capable of reducing both pain AND swelling following surgery.

In regards to pain and swelling, you can only imagine how effective cold laser is for common sprains and strains and other musculoskeletal complaints that chiropractors see every day[119].

EFFECTIVENESS OF COLD LASER THERAPY

Here's some research that demonstrates cold laser's effectiveness as a treatment for pain.

This one is called "The effectiveness of low-level laser therapy for nonspecific chronic low back pain: a systematic review and meta-analysis." It was done in 2015 and published in Arthritis Research & Therapy.

Why They Did It

With low back pain being the cause of such a large percentage of doctor and emergency room visits, healthcare researchers are steadily searching for new and effective means for treating it. Cold laser therapy has enjoyed some solid research in the past, but its effectiveness for treating nonspecific chronic low back pain (NSCLBP) has seen some conflicting results.

How They Did It
- The authors systematically searched databases (MEDLINE, EMBASE, ISI Web of Science, and Cochrane Library).
- They only used results from January 2000-November 2014.
- 221 studies were reviewed and only 7 were accepted for this paper.

- The studies accepted for this review used randomized controlled trials that compared low level laser therapy (cold laser therapy) with placebo for treatment of nonspecific chronic low back pain.

What They Found
- Using the common pain measurement called the visual analog scale (VAS), it was determined that the average pain score following treatments with cold laser was significantly lower when compared to the placebo group average.
- No determination could be made on effectiveness for disability scores or range of motion results.

Wrap It Up
There was no determination on whether cold laser can help with function or lack thereof. However, the authors found, and concluded, that low-level laser therapy, or cold laser therapy, is indeed effective in treating patients suffering from nonspecific chronic low back pain[120].

COLD LASER FOR ARTHRITIC KNEE PAIN - DOES IT WORK?

Considering the that many times our knees fail as we age and the number of knee replacement surgeries continues to rise, it is important to find a way to reduce symptoms to alleviate knee discomfort.

This paper shows some real promise for Cold Laser therapy, also known as Low Level Laser (LLL). This study is for osteoarthritis of the knee alone. However, Cold Laser therapy is useful in the treatment of MANY complaints such as sprains or strains, inflammation, and pain in general. It's so effective that professional sports teams are employing its use every day. It's top-of-the-line treatment for their athletes.

Jeff S. Williams, DC, FIANM

Why They Did It

Osteoarthritis (OA) is more and more common in elderly and commonly leads to disability. Can Cold Laser help to either avoid surgery or lessen the symptoms?

How They Did It
- 18 patients with osteoarthritis in the knee
- They were treated with LLL three times a week for 12 sessions
- Patient results were tracked using SPSS ver. 15.

What They Found
- A clinically significant reduction was seen regarding pain at night.
- A clinically significant reduction was seen regarding pain while walking.
- A clinically significant reduction was seen regarding pain while going up stairs.
- A clinically significant reduction in the size of the knee.

Wrap It Up

The authors reported that Cold Laser (LLL) was in fact effective in reducing pain in knee osteoarthritis[121].

COLD LASER AND TMJ. WHAT DOES THE RESEARCH SAY?

More and more health practitioners are beginning to recognize the benefits of cold laser or low-level laser (LLL). More and more research continues to validate the trend and in response, we are seeing increased utilization across the board. Here is a short research paper having to do with the efficacy of LLL on temporomandibular disorders (TMJ) (TMD).

Why They Did It

Considering it's "newness" as a healthcare treatment option, LLL still needs more and more research to validate its usefulness and efficacy across a wide spectrum of conditions and complaints. This study was to confirm the efficacy of red and infrared laser therapy for TMJ disorders.

How They Did It

- Most importantly, the trial was a DOUBLE-BLIND, RANDOMIZED, parallel clinical trial.
- Each TMJ joint of 19 subjects was randomized in a total of 116 points
- Pain was measured at 24 hours, 30 days, 90 days, and 180 days after treatment
- There were 3 sessions of treatment

What They Found

- Both the red and the infrared LLL had significant results.
- There was a difference between the two treatments at 180 days with the infrared being the more effective.
- There was improvement from 24 hours all the way to the 180-day mark for both laser treatment types.

Wrap It Up

Both infrared and red cold laser (LLL) showed to be significantly effective in a double-blind, randomized parallel clinical trial for the treatment of temporomandibular joint disorder (TMJ) (TMD)[122].

A COUPLE OF WAYS TO DECREASE YOUR NECK PAIN

Here's a study from 2011 about neck pain treatment. It's a randomized controlled study showing the effectiveness of cervical manipulation and cold laser (low level laser) treatment for facet dysfunction.

Why They Did It

The goal was to find out the effectiveness of cervical manipulation combined with cold laser for the treatment of cervical facet syndrome. This condition is a common trigger for neck pain in otherwise healthy individuals.

How They Did It

- 6 women were accepted into the study.
- Their ages ranged between 18 and 40 yrs old.
- They all suffered from cervical facet joint pain lasting more than 30 days.
- Their treatments were randomized into 3 different protocol groups:
  - Manipulation (Chiropractic)
  - Cold laser
  - A combination of the two treatments
- The following Outcome Assessments were used to measure the results and effectiveness:
  - Numeric Pain Rating Scale
  - Neck Disability Index
  - Cervical Range of Motion Instrument
  - Baseline Digital Inclinometer
- Measurements were taken in weeks 1, 2, 3, and 4.

What They Found

Significant improvements were found among all treatment groups, but the improvements were most noticeable with group three.

Wrap It Up

All three groups showed improvement, but a combination of manipulation and cold laser proved most effective. Both are proven to be viable treatment protocols for cervical facet syndrome[62]

PREGNANCY

POWERFUL RESEARCH ON PREGNANCY-INDUCED PAIN AND CHIROPRACTIC CARE

Why They Did It

A very common complaint in pregnancy is low back pain. No question about it. The authors of this paper wanted to test the theory: is a multimodal approach to treating the pregnancy-induced low back pain more effective than standard and usual OBGYN care?

How They Did It

- This study was a prospective, randomized trial.
- 169 subjects were accepted for inclusion.
- A baseline assessment was performed on the patients at the 24-28-week gestation period.
- The assessment was followed up with another assessment at the 33-week mark.
- The Numerical Rating Scale (NRS) was used to assess pain for each patient.
- The Quebec Disability Rating (QRS) was used as well for pain assessment.
- Each of the 2 groups received routine OBGYN care.
- In one of the groups however, chiropractors treated the women with manual therapy, stabilization exercises, and patient education.

What They Found

In the group in which Chiropractic was utilized, a significant reduction in pain was reported by the patients from baseline to finish.

The regular OBGYN group had no significant improvement.

Wrap It Up

"A multimodal approach to low back and pelvic pain in mid pregnancy benefits patients more than standard obstetric care[123]."

PREGNANCY, LOW BACK PAIN, CHIROPRACTIC NEW RESEARCH

Why They Did It

With low back pain being so predominant in pregnant women, the authors noticed that research on pregnancy and chiropractic was fairly limited. They saw the need to
- Report the results that women got from chiropractic treatment during pregnancy.
- To compare those results to the outcomes from subgroups
- To investigate whether there are ways to predict the outcomes

How They Did It
- Patients had to be pregnant and have low back or pelvic pain.
- They could not have contraindications to manipulative therapy.
- They could not have had any manual therapy for three months prior to the treatments.
- Factors such as low back pain during a previous pregnancy, category of pain, duration of complaint, and number of previous episodes were all recorded and tracked.
- They used several factors to record the Outcome Assessments for these patients and performed the Outcome Assessments at 1 week, 1 month, 3 months, 6 months, and 1-year post treatment.
- The patient's global impression of change was measured. (PGIC)

- The Numeric Rating System was utilized as well – estimating pain on a scale from 1-10
- Oswestry Questionnaire

What They Found
- 52% of 115 recruited patients 'improved' at 1 week,
- 70% at 1 month,
- 85% at 3 months,
- 90% at 6 months and
- 88% at 1 year.

Wrap Up.
The majority of pregnant chiropractic patients with low back pain that underwent chiropractic treatment showed clinically relevant improvement, results, and recovery at all time points that the Outcome Assessments were performed[124].

NEW FINDINGS FOR MANIPULATIVE THERAPY IN PREGNANCY

WHY THEY DID IT
The reason for this paper was to test the effectiveness of manipulative techniques during pregnancy for the treatment of back and pelvic pain.

HOW THEY DID IT
- It was based on a review of available literature through a MEDLINE and a Cochrane Library search in January of 2014
- They looked for relevant reports, randomized controlled trials, and case studies.
- Each source was verified and analyzed.

WHAT THEY FOUND

After an exhaustive search and analysis of the literature, the authors concluded that manipulative protocols appear effective and safe in pregnant women for low back and pelvic pain[125].

A POWERFUL WAY TO ADDRESS
YOUR PAIN DURING PREGNANCY

Why They Did It

The goal was to outline the chiropractic management of a prenatal patient experiencing lumbopelvic pain.

How They Did It

- The paper is a simple case report.
- The patient was 35 years old and suffered from moderate to severe lumbopelvic pain directly related to her pregnancy.
- The patient also suffered associated leg pain.
- The patient was limited in her ability to walk and sit.
- Her complaint, through an exam, was determined to be brought on by dysfunction of the left sacroiliac joint with associated back and leg pain.
- Chiropractic manipulations were used to treat the condition as well as soft tissue therapy, postural correction, and exercise.
- The patient has thirteen appointments over a period of 6 weeks.
- She visited with her OBGYN simultaneously and weekly.

What They Found

- The patient's lumbopelvic complaint improved significantly from a 7 to a 2 using the Numeric Rating Scale (NRS).
- In addition, activities of daily living were much improved (walking, sitting, etc..)

Wrap It Up

Significant improvement was seen in this case study through the use of Chiropractic, manual therapy, and exercise[126].

A SUCCESSFUL TREATMENT FOR LOW BACK PAIN IN PREGNANCY

Why They Did It

With low back complaints being so prevalent in expectant mothers, the goal of this paper was to add to the literature regarding pregnancy-related low back pain and chiropractic manipulation as a treatment option. Knowing that chiropractic manipulation is proven to be effective in low back pain, the authors wanted to explore the results of chiropractic treatment for a group of pregnant patients having low back pain as a result of the pregnancy.

How They Did It

- Data showed that as few as 32% of patients reported symptoms to their healthcare provider.
- Only 25% of the healthcare providers actually recommended treatment for the symptoms.
- The study was a retrospective case series.
- 17 patients were accepted into the study.
- They performed self-assessment using the Numeric Ratings System (NRS).

What They Found

- The average NRS score was reduces from a 5.9 all the way down to a 1.5 average at the ending of the care plan.
- 94.1% of the patients showed clinically important improvement.
- On average, it took the patients an average of 4 1/2 days to achieve clinically significant pain relief.
- On average, it took roughly 2 visits to achieve the

improvement.
- NO adverse effects were experienced by any of the subjects.

Wrap It Up
"The results suggest that chiropractic treatment was safe in these cases and support the hypothesis that it may be effective for reducing pain intensity[127]."

A HELPFUL WAY TO EXPLORE CHIROPRACTIC FOR PREGNANCY PAINS

Why They Did It
There have been several studies showing the efficacy of chiropractic treatment for low back pain. However, there have been none exploring the EXPERIENCE itself. The authors of this paper wanted to try to fill that hole in the research literature.

How They Did It
- This was a qualitative study.
- This paper used semi-structured question and answer sessions with the subjects.
- The patients needed to be in their second or third trimester and be suffering from pregnancy-induced low back pain to qualify for inclusion in the study.
- The interviews were conducted with the patients as well as the chiropractors involved.
- The questions had to do with topics such as what their experience was during treatment, etc.
- The interviews were reviewed and analyzed independently.

What They Found

Jeff S. Williams, DC, FIANM

- From the interviews, five themes were noticed.
- The themes were as follows:
  - i) Treatment & Effectiveness
  - ii) Chiropractor-Patient Communication
  - iii) Pregnant Patient Presentation and the Chiropractic Approach to Pregnancy Care
  - iv) Safety Considerations
  - v) Self-Care

Wrap It Up

"Chiropractors approach pregnant patients with low back pain from a patient-centered standpoint, and the pregnant patients interviewed in this study who sought chiropractic care appeared to find this approach helpful for managing their back pain symptoms[128]."

Jeff S. Williams, DC, FIANM

CAR WRECK INJURIES & WHIPLASH

This section could fill an entire textbook. In fact, it has. For more information on whiplash, chiropractic management of car wreck injuries, and its efficacy, one of the premier authorities in the nation is Dr. Arthur Croft with the Spine Research Institute of San Diego. He has written the textbook. Actually, he has written several of them I believe.

I have a couple of reasons for including this section in this book:
1. The blogs have already been written so why not include them?
2. The information backing chiropractic comes in many shapes and sizes. If we have great information, it should be shared and shared again.

The amount of research in chiropractic's favor regarding whiplash and car wreck injury is simply too robust to adequately address here.

If you are hungry for more, again, please consult Dr. Arthur Croft of the SPINE Institute in San Diego, CA.

HOW EFFECTIVE IS CHIROPRACTIC FOR WHIPLASH INJURIES

Before we get into the research too heavily, I would like to make the following points:
- Patients: Be certain you are going to a practitioner that truly has experience in the treatment of personal injury and

has done the work required to be proficient in your case management.
- Practitioners: Do the work and get the knowledge you need to do your personal injury patients justice. All it takes to mess up their case or its management, is a small amount of ignorance. You must always be at the forefront to do it right.

I have seen some amazing turn-arounds in the world of whiplash. Whiplash symptoms are varied; however, the most common symptoms are neck pain, mid-back pain, headaches, and numbness or pain into the arms.

Here's a research paper on just how effective chiropractic treatment can be for this sort of injury.

Why They Did It
To attempt to determine what type of whiplash patient would be the ones that would respond the best to chiropractic treatment.

How They Did It
- The study took 100 patients with chronic pain due to whiplash
- Seven fell out of the study
- 93 patients made up the final group
- 25 were male and 68 were female
- Patients received an average of 19.3 adjustments throughout roughly 4 months of treatment
- They were divided into three distinct groups
  Group 1: Neck pain radiating into the shoulders, restricted range of neck movement but no neurological issues.
  Group 2: Neurological symptoms (pain or numbness into arms) with neck discomfort and decreased range of motion.
  Group 3: A mishmash of symptoms such as blackouts, visual disturbances, sleep disturbances, etc. Also having neck pain described as severe but a full range of motion and no neurological signs.

Jeff S. Williams, DC, FIANM

- Group 1: 72% improved. 24% becoming asymptomatic and 24% improving by two symptom grades.
- Group 2. 94% responded positively. 38% became asymptomatic while 43% improved by 2 symptom grades.
- Group 3: 27% of these patients improved. All stayed symptomatic.

Wrap It Up

The authors of the paper concluded "The results from this study provide further evidence that chiropractic is an effective treatment for chronic whiplash symptoms[129]."

STEPPING OFF OF A CURB IS NOT THE SAME THING

"Is Acceleration a Valid Proxy for Injury Risk in Minimal Damage Traffic Crashes? A Comparative Review of Volunteer, ADL and Real-World Studies" by Nolet, et. al. [130] published in International Journal of Environmental Research and Public Health in March of 2021.

Why They Did It

Let me preface this by saying that Dr. Michael Freeman is an author on this paper and he's just a phenomenal asset to chiropractic, health in general, and personal injury research. If you aren't familiar with Dr. Freeman, we're talking about the fact that he's a DC, an MD, and Ph.D. and a whole bunch of other stuff one single person has any business being.

Also on this paper is Dr. Art Croft. I have the advanced certification through Dr. Croft's SPINE Institute in San Diego and I have to tell you that he's one of the most impressive individuals I've ever personally met.

In the paper, they say, "Injury claims associated with minimal damage rear impact traffic crashes are often defended using a "biomechanical approach," in which the occupant forces of the crash are compared to the forces of activities of daily living (ADLs), resulting in the conclusion that the risk of injury from the crash is the same as for ADLs. The purpose of the present investigation is to evaluate the scientific validity of the central operating premise of the biomechanical approach to injury causation; that occupant acceleration is a scientifically valid proxy for injury risk."

How They Did It
- Data were abstracted, pooled, and compared from three categories of published literature:
    1. Volunteer rear-impact crash testing studies,
    2. ADL studies, and
    3. Observational studies of real-world rear impacts.
    - We compared the occupant accelerations of minimal or no damage (i.e., 3 to 11 kph speed change or "delta-V") (2 mph up to 7 mph.) rear-impact crash tests to the accelerations described in 6 of the **most commonly reported ADLs in the reviewed studies.**
    - As a final step, the injury risk observed in real-world crashes was compared to the results of the pooled crash test and ADL analyses, controlling for delta-V.
    - OK in me and you speak, Delta V just means the change in speed that was experienced. Anytime you are in a wreck, you essentially go from one speed to another in a millisecond. That's not conceptually, that's literally. Delta V helps to describe that change in speed.

What They Found
- The results of the analyses indicated that average peak acceleration forces observed at the head during rear impact crash tests were typically at least several times greater than average forces observed during activities of daily living.

- In contrast, the injury risk of real-world minimal damage rear impact crashes was estimated to be at least 2000 times greater than for any activities of daily living.

Wrap It Up

"The results of our analysis indicate that the principle underlying the biomechanical injury causation approach, that occupant acceleration is a proxy for injury risk, is scientifically invalid. The biomechanical approach to injury causation in minimal damage crashes invariably results in the vast underestimation of the actual risk of such crashes and should be discontinued as it is a scientifically invalid practice."

NECK INJURIES IN CAR WRECKS IS MORE COMMON THAN THEY WANT YOU TO THINK

"Estimating the number of traffic crash-related cervical spine injuries in the United States; An analysis and comparison of national crash and hospital data" by Michael Freeman and Wendy Leith [131] and published in Accident Analysis And Prevention in July of 2020 and that's still got some steam to it.

Why They Did It

In the intro, they say, "Cervical spine injury is a common result of traffic crashes, and such injuries range in severity from minor (i.e. sprain/strain) to moderate (intervertebral disk derangement) to serious and greater (fractures, dislocations, and spinal cord injuries). There are currently no reliable estimates of the number of crash-related spine injuries occurring in the US annually, although several publications have used national crash injury samples as a basis for estimating the frequency of both cervical and lumbar spinal disk injuries occurring in lower speed rear impact crashes. To develop a reliable estimate of the number of various types of cervical spine injuries occurring in the US by comparing data from national crash injury to national hospital emergency departments and inpatient samples."

How They Did It

Comparative cross-sectional METHODS: Cervical spine injury data were accessed, analyzed, and compared from 3 national databases; the

1. National Automotive Sampling System-Crashworthiness Data System (NASS-CDS),
2. Nationwide Emergency Department Sample (NEDS), and the
3. Nationwide Inpatient Sample (NIS).

What They Found

- It is estimated that there are approximately 869,000 traffic crash-related cervical spine injuries seen in hospitals in the US annually, including around
  - 841,000 sprain/strain (whiplash) injuries,
  - 2800 spinal disk injuries,
  - 23,500 fractures,
  - 2800 spinal cord injuries, and
  - 1500 dislocations.
- Because of highly restrictive inclusion criteria for both crash and injury types, as well as a very small sample size, the NASS-CDS underestimated all types of crash-related cervical spine injuries seen in US hospital emergency departments by 84 %
- The injury type with the largest degree of underestimation in the NASS-CDS was cervical disk injuries, which were estimated at an 88 % lower frequency than in the Nationwide Emergency Department Sample
- National insurance claim data, which include cases of cervical disk injury diagnosed both in and outside of the ED, indicate that the Nationwide Emergency Department Sample likely undercounts cervical disk injuries by 92 %, and thus the NASS-CDS correspondingly undercounts such injuries by 99 % or more.

Wrap It Up

They end it by saying "Because of a limited sample size and restrictive criteria for both crash and injury inclusion, the NASS-CDS cannot be used to estimate the number of crash-related spinal injuries of any type or severity in the US. The most inappropriate use of the database is for estimating the number of spinal injuries resulting from low-speed rear impact collisions, as the NASS-CDS samples fewer than 1 in 100,000 of the cervical spine injuries of any type occurring in low-speed rear impact collisions."

A SURGING SOLUTION FOR WHIPLASH INJURIES

Why They Did It

The goal of the paper was to basically pit chiropractic manipulative therapy against physiotherapy for treatment of whiplash injuries. Which would be more effective?

How They Did It

- This paper was a randomized controlled trial.
- 380 volunteers were accepted into the study.
- 300 of them were males, 80 were female.
- All patients had been diagnosed with whiplash injuries less than 3 months old.
- The Whiplash gradings were in the Grade II to Grade III range using the Quebec Task Force grading system.
- The patients were divided randomly into 2 groups. Group A was the experimental group while Group B was the control group.
- Group A underwent a manipulative (chiropractic) regimen with weekly adjustments and included soft tissue manipulation and mobilization.
- Group B underwent traditional physiotherapy/physical therapy protocols daily which included active exercise, electrotherapy, ultrasound, and diathermy.

- The Outcome Assessments were performed via the Visual Analogue Scale (VAS), the cervical range of motion, and amount of treatment required to finish the protocol.
- The data was run at the beginning, after each 4 session for the first group and after every 10th session in the second (control) group.

What They Found
- In the chiropractic group, the patients needed an average of 9 visits to complete treatment.
- In the physiotherapy group, the patients needed an average of 23 sessions.
- The chiropractic group had much more improvement than did the physiotherapy group in the Outcome Assessments, particularly after the first 4 sessions.

Wrap It Up
"Patients who had received manipulative treatment needed fewer sessions to complete the treatment than patients who had received physiotherapy treatment. The improvement in the manipulative group was achieved with fewer treatment sessions and was greater than the improvement in physiotherapy group[132]."

Can Pre-Existing Risk Factors Affect A Whiplash Injury?

Here is some research that explores the impact of pre-existing factors on one's injuries following a motor vehicle crash.

Why They Did It
- Figure out what risk factors people had that caused chronic disability following whiplash injuries.
- Attempt to understand the impact of those risk factors on them.

How They Did It

- Reports were collected approximately thirty-two days after the traumatic injury and then again twelve months later.
- There were baseline measurements collected in regard to disability, neck movement/range of motion, pain, psychological and behavioral indicators, as well as chronic disability at the 12-month mark.
- The main way to measure outcomes was through the use of the Neck Disability Index Questionnaire

What They Found

- Psychological and Behavioral factors were important when considering chronic disability following a whiplash injury.
- The number of risk factors involved in the incident is important when evaluating patients and their likely outcomes following whiplash[133].

MORE THAN HALF SUSTAIN LONG-LASTING SYMPTOMS FROM CAR WRECKS

Why They Did It

The idea was to evaluate patient use of sick leave in the years following a car wreck and to determine how much of that sick leave could be attributed to the car wreck.

How They Did It

- For a period of time, from 1985-1990, Borchgrevink et. al. did a review of car wreck cases that were seen through the Emergency Clinic at The University Hospital in Trondheim, Norway.
- There were 426 patients seen during that period of time with neck sprain injuries after car wrecks.
- 345 of the patients filled out the questionnaire having to do with quality of life following the wreck, plus a review of information from the Trondheim Social Security office was performed.

What They Found
- 27% of the people had reported taking sick leave during the time just following the accident.
- 58% reported sustained symptoms that were linked directly to the accident itself. This is important since car insurance companies try to tell us that soft tissue injuries heal after only 3-6 weeks.
- 16% reported being in a bad state of health.

Wrap It Up
As mentioned above, insurance companies may try to reduce payment on car wreck victims' health bills due to a misguided notion that all soft tissue heals in 3-6 weeks. This is absolutely false.

If a muscle alone were strained, then yes, it should heal within that time frame since muscle is well-organized, well-vascularized, and heals more rapidly.

However, if ligaments or tendons are sprained in the collision, which is more the rule than the exception, the damage can be long-lasting and potentially chronic. It could potentially last a lifetime.

This study is important as it definitely hints at the potential chronic nature of car wrecks in even mild collisions [134].

A SIMPLE AND POWERFUL WAY TO ADDRESS NECK PAIN

Why They Did It
The authors of this paper wished to find out if conservative therapies like manual therapy, mobilization, etc. are effective for function and/or disability and patient happiness, as well as other factors.

Jeff S. Williams, DC, FIANM

How They Did It

- 11 systematic reviews consisting of randomized controlled trials were updated.
- The studies were chosen for inclusion in this paper by 2 independent reviewers.
- Relative risks and standardized mean differences were calculated.
- 88 unique randomized controlled trials were studied.

What They Found

- There was strong evidence that pain was reduced, function was improved, and there was a positive global perceived effect in regard to manipulation and exercise over the control group.
- There was moderate evidence that neck strengthening and stretching were effective for chronic neck disorders.
- There was zero evidence for botulinium-A injection.

Wrap It Up

"Exercise combined with mobilization/manipulation demonstrated either intermediate or long-term benefits[135]."

A POWERFUL & STRONG FINDING FOR WHIPLASH INJURY TREATMENT

Why They Did It

Whiplash is a common malady following motor vehicle crashes. The authors of this paper estimate 43% of crash victims will go on to experience long-term suffering from whiplash injuries. The authors wanted to explore the efficacy of chiropractic treatment in such complaints.

- The study was a retrospective study.
- Chronic whiplash patients were accepted into the study.
- The chiropractic treatment group consisted of 28 patients.
- The severity of the whiplash injury was assessed at the baseline via the Gargan & Bannister classification system.

What They Found
- 93% of the test subjects improved after undergoing the chiropractic protocol.

Wrap It Up

The results of this study were so promising and favorable for chiropractic treatment in whiplash that the authors felt a randomized controlled trial comparing this treatment with convention treatment was warranted to explore it further[136].

AN IMPROVED APPROACH FOR WHIPLASH INJURY TREATMENT

Why They Did It

Since there was a vacuum in the literature concerning the frequency and efficacy of thoracic manipulation in whiplash cases, the goal of this paper was to determine efficacy of thoracic manipulation in that context.

How They Did It

There were two parts to the study.
1. The first part of the study consisted of:
   - 120 patients having mechanical neck pain
   - 120 patient diagnosed with whiplash
     - The question was tested: Are there any differences in the prevalence of thoracic joint dysfunction between patients diagnosed with mechanical neck pain and those diagnosed with having whiplash?

2. The second part consisted of:
   - 88 patients from the initial 120.
   - These 88 were divided randomly into 2 groups (Group A and Group B)
   - Group A was the experimental group
   - Group B was the control group
   - Group A underwent treatment consisting of thoracic manipulation and physiotherapy techniques. The adjustments occurred at the 5th visit and at the 10th visit.
   - Group B underwent treatment consisting of only physiotherapy techniques.
   - Outcome Assessment included the visual analog scale (VAS).
   - Data was collected before treatment commenced, after the 10th session, and after the 15th session.

What They Found

- They found that in the first section of the study 69% of those diagnosed with whiplash also had thoracic dysfunction.
- Only 13% with mechanical neck pain had associated thoracic dysfunction.
- For the other part of the paper, the experimental group (chiropractic adjustment group) had a more significant reduction in their VAS score than did the physiotherapy alone group.
- This difference was most noticeable in the intensity of neck pain after the second adjustment and in back pain after the 1st and 2nd adjustments.

Wrap It Up

Thoracic dysfunction occurs frequently (roughly 70% of the time) in conjunction with whiplash injury, and chiropractic manipulation combined with exercise and therapy is more beneficial than exercise and therapy alone[137].

Jeff S. Williams, DC, FIANM

INTEGRATED APPROACH

CAN A COMBINED MEDICAL AND CHIROPRACTIC APPROACH WORK?

There has been much more research surfacing lately regarding an INTEGRATED practice offering a COMBINED treatment protocol for musculoskeletal complaints.

Meaning, if your neck hurts, rather than only going to the medical doctor and getting pain killers, muscle relaxers, and/or anti-inflammatories, you would go to a chiropractor in addition to the traditional medical treatment regimen.

Why They Did It
This research from 2011 explored a hospital-based standardized spine care treatment pathway, including the results of the multidisciplinary protocol.

How They Did It
- They used 518 patients
- They developed a standard Spine Care Pathway treatment protocol
- The National Center for Quality Assurance (NCQA) back pain recognition program (BPRP) was used as the framework for the Spine Care Pathway
- Patients were categorized based on several factors.
- 83% of the patients qualified for and underwent chiropractic care and/or physical therapy.

- Those that also attended treatment with a Doctor of Chiropractic attended about 5.2 visits at a cost of about $302.
- On intake, the pain rating score was 6.2 out of 10.
- On exit, the pain rating was 1.9 out of 10.
- Of the patients also attending chiropractic treatment, 95% of them rated their care as EXCELLENT.

Wrap It Up

A combined, integrated treatment protocol proved less expensive and achieved higher patient satisfaction upon completion[138].

ARE CHIROPRACTORS GREEDY & EXPENSIVE?

A misperception I hear from time to time is that chiropractors are greedy or just want to see how many times they can get a patient in and out of their doors purely for financial gain.

Let's not beat around the bush: there most certainly are opportunists in EVERY profession in the world. I'm certain that chiropractic is no exception. So, every now and then, they may be right.

However, people in general are good by nature, and again chiropractors are no exception. Truly, the vast majority of chiropractors got into business for no other reason than to help people.

Before we dive into the research, ask yourself a simple question, "If my primary sent me to a physical therapist, would they just see me once and tell me to call if it keeps bothering me?" If you've had any experience with physical therapy, you already know the answer to that question. Of course not! You'll be treated on a steady and consistent basis for a specific amount of time, because any change in the body or substantial healing takes time and consistency.

In addition, building durability to avoid future worsening of the original injury is something that takes work. This is mostly common sense.

With that being said, let's dive in. The Manga Report is an old chiropractic stand-by. This report has been around for some time now.

It's been around since 1993 to be exact.

Why They Did It
To assess the effectiveness in terms of physical recovery or pain alleviation, as well as the cost-effectiveness of chiropractic, in regard to treating low back pain.

How They Did It
The Ontario Ministry of Health-commissioned study was a comprehensive review of all of the published literature on low back pain.

What They Found
- They found an overwhelming amount of evidence showing the effectiveness of chiropractic in the treatment of low back pain.
- They also found that chiropractic care is more cost-effective than traditional medical treatment and management.
- Found that many of the traditional medical therapies used in low back pain are considered questionable in validity, and while some are very safe, others can lead to more problems for the patient.
- There are no case controlled studies that suggest that chiropractic is unsafe for the treatment of low back pain. They clearly showed that chiropractic is more cost-effective and there would be highly significant savings if more low back pain management was controlled by chiropractors rather than medical physicians.

- The study stated that chiropractic services should be fully insured.
- The study stated that services should be fully integrated into the overall healthcare system due to the high cost of low back pain and the cost-effectiveness and physical effectiveness of chiropractic.
- They also stated that a good case could be made for making chiropractors the entry point into the healthcare system for musculoskeletal complaints that presented to hospitals.

Wrap It Up
Chiropractic should be the treatment of choice for low back pain, even excluding traditional medical care altogether[21]!

EXPERT PROOF FOR LOW BACK PAIN TREATMENT RECOMMENDATIONS

Why They Did It
The authors in this paper note that low back pain is the 5th most prevalent issue causing people to seek treatment at a doctor's office. They go on to state that about 25% of Americans adults experienced low back pain lasting an entire day at least one time in the previous three months. In addition, low back pain cost about $26.3 billion back in 1998.

The authors wanted to conduct a systematic review of the available evidence regarding the treatment of low back pain in adults.

How They Did It
- Data was collected via literature taken from sources such as MEDLINE, Cochrane Database of Systematic Reviews, the Cochrane Central Register of Controlled Trials, and EMBASE.
- The papers only contained randomized, controlled trials on patients having low back pain (with or without associated leg pain).

Jeff S. Williams, DC, FIANM

- The patients needed to have reported at least 1 of the following Outcome Assessments:
back-specific function
generic health status
pain
work disability
patient satisfaction
- The American College of Physicians and the American Pain Society collaborated to create guidelines and procedures for the review and subsequent recommendations.

What They Found
- "For acute low back pain (duration <4 weeks), spinal manipulation administered by providers with appropriate training is associated with small to moderate short-term benefits.
- For chronic low back pain, moderately effective non-pharmacologic therapies include acupuncture, exercise therapy, massage therapy, Viniyoga-style yoga, cognitive-behavioral therapy or progressive relaxation, spinal manipulation, and intensive interdisciplinary rehabilitation."

Wrap It Up
Complementary and Alternative Medicine (CAM) protocols are absolutely effective for both long-term and acute low back pain and should be considered as an entry point into the healthcare system for mechanical low back pain[43].

COST-EFFECTIVENESS

CHIROPRACTIC MORE COST-EFFECTIVE AND MORE EFFECTIVE OVERALL THAN GENERAL PRACTITIONER

Why They Did It

The authors of this paper wished to perform a review of trial-based economic evaluations that have been performed for manual therapy in comparison to other treatment protocols used for treatment of musculoskeletal complaints.

How They Did It
- The authors performed a comprehensive literature search of commonly used research databases for all subjects relative to this subject.
- 25 publications were included.
- The studies included cost-effectiveness for manual therapies compared to other forms of treatment for pain.

What They Found
- Manual therapy techniques such as chiropractic mobilization were more cost effective than visiting a general practitioner.
- Specifically, chiropractic treatment was less costly and was found to be more effective than physiotherapy/physical therapy or visiting a general practitioner's medical office when treating neck pain.

Wrap It Up

Although improvement in our knowledge of manual therapies is warranted, this paper demonstrates that chiropractic is more cost-effective and more effective in general for low back pain & shoulder disability than usual medical practitioner care and physical therapy/physiotherapy[25].

ARE YOU SPENDING TOO MUCH ON THAT NECK PAIN?

This paper shows that it makes more financial sense to seek out a chiropractor for neuro-musculoskeletal issues before consulting our medical counterparts.

This article is from 2016, so it is current and relevant.

Why They Did It

The authors wanted to compare how services were used and charged in the healthcare field by doctors of chiropractic and medical doctors.

How They Did It

- They used data from 2000 to 2009 from North Carolina State Health Plan for Teachers and State Employees (NCSHP).
- They used diagnostic codes for uncomplicated neck pain as well as complicated neck pain.

What They Found

- Single providers that did not refer their patients to others racked up the least in charges on average for both uncomplicated neck pain as well as complicated pain.
- When care did not include referrals, medical doctor care with physical therapy was generally less expensive than medical care and chiropractic care combined.

- treatment protocols including referral providers, medical doctor care, and physical therapist care was more expensive on the average than medical care combined with chiropractic care for either condition.
- Charges for chiropractic patients in the middle quintiles of risk had lower bills with or without medical care or referral care to other providers.

Wrap It Up

Chiropractic care alone OR chiropractic care in combination with medical care had significantly lower charges for uncomplicated neck pain or complicated neck pain when compared to medical care with or without physical therapy care[34].

A HIGHER PURPOSE

WHY I WROTE THIS BOOK - THE BIGGER MISSION

The answer to the question of why I wrote this book is multifactorial.
1. I wanted an easy-to-find, quick reference for tracking down research for presentations or self- and patient-education purposes. I assumed that if I would find value in such a resource, so would my colleagues.
2. I want to change certain aspects of the chiropractic profession. Certain aspects of the community that I have been troubled by since I was in school.

The first objective is self-explanatory so I will focus more on the second one.

As the writer and host of The Chiropractic Forward Podcast, every effort has been made by me to continually and consistently advocate evidence-based, patient-centered care.

If you have made it this far in the book, then I would like to invite you to first, PLEASE go REVIEW this book on Amazon. Your review boosts the book up the charts, which boosts sales, which expands the message of evidence-based, patient-centered chiropractic.

Next I would like to invite you to join us online and join me by listening to The Chiropractic Forward Podcast each week. A new episode typically posts every Thursday. Each episode is full and includes personal happenings and business struggles, sometimes we have movers and shakers in the profession join us for interviews, and it always includes 2-4 research papers pertinent to the chiropractic profession in one way or another.

Here are some relevant links for you to find us and engage:

> Chiropractic Forward Podcast & Online Store
> http://www.chiropracticforward.com

> Chiropractic Forward Podcast Facebook PAGE
> https://www.facebook.com/chiropracticforward/

> Chiropractic Forward Podcast Facebook GROUP
> https://www.facebook.com/groups/1938461399501889/

> Chiropractic Forward Twitter
> https://twitter.com/Chiro_Forward

> Chiropractic Forward YouTube Channel
> www.youtube.com/channel/UCtc-IrhlK19hWlhaOGld76Q

> Chiropractic Forward RSS link
> https://www.chiropracticforward.com/rss

> Chiropractic Forward iTunes Link:
> https://podcasts.apple.com/us/podcast/chiropractic-forward-podcast-evidence-based-chiropractic/id1331554445

> Chiropractic Forward Player FM Link
> https://player.fm/series/2291021

> Chiropractic Forward Stitcher Link:
> https://www.stitcher.com/podcast/the-chiropractic-forward-podcast-chiropractors-practicing-through

> Chiropractic Forward TuneIn Link
> https://tunein.com/podcasts/Health--Wellness-Podcasts/The-Chiropractic-Forward-Podcast-Chiropractors-Pr-p1089415/

To close out this book, I want to share with you some thoughts on characteristics and qualities I look for in a good chiropractor.

I saw a question on social media. The question was about what qualities we look for in other chiropractors before we'll recommend them to a family member or to a friend.

Quite honestly, I get phone calls, text messages, Facebook messages, and emails from friends and associates that live out of town asking

Jeff S. Williams, DC, FIANM

me if I know a good chiropractor where they live. I get these requests literally all of the time. And if I don't know one, then what is the best way to choose a chiropractor?

I think that any time one decides that they're going to go to a new doctor....even for you and for me.....if we change doctors, there is a certain amount of apprehension. In choosing a chiropractor, this apprehension can be escalated to a certain extent because all chiropractors are vastly different. In short, there is literally zero standardization in the profession. It's like the wild wild West out there in some aspects.

For example, if you have an ear infection and you go to the ED, you know it's going to be a pretty standard treatment, right? Not so with chiropractic. You can go in for a little tweak in your back and walk out $3500 lighter with a year long plan for care that research does not support the need for. Or you can walk in with a little tweak in your back and get some completely normal, responsible recommendation.

Let's be fair though, this is not a problem that is specific to only chiropractic. My wife has had several dentists over the years try to put one over on her for thousands and thousands of dollars. It is not as much a profession problem as it is a 'people problem' in my estimation. Still, the chiropractic profession has far too much of it present within.

There are some chiropractors that focus on weight loss. There are some chiropractors that only use an instrument to adjust rather than manual adjusting.

There are some chiropractors that are more driven by philosophy than other chiropractors. There are some chiropractors that use therapy and extra equipment, while other chiropractors only adjust and have refused to update their thinking through the years as research and knowledge has passed them by. The good news about that is that there is indeed a chiropractor for every different type of person and preference. The bad news about that is that they are not all good and, it is my opinion, that a healthcare profession should evolve as the research literature progresses and the knowledge base expands.

Chiropractic, for many, stays frozen in their minds, behavior, thought processes, and treatment. It stays frozen back in the late 1800's when the profession was first formulated.

Keeping it all in mind, let's dive into 9 characteristics I feel are important in a good chiropractor.

HONESTY

Other than the first topic and the last topic, I have not put these qualities in any specific order. But I put honesty at the top of the pile because I feel strongly about it.

I feel that honesty is of utmost importance in any profession. Especially in the healthcare field. People are literally putting their lives and their livelihoods in our hands. You would like to think our family is putting their lives in the hands of an honest person, wouldn't you think?

We've heard it said time and time again that if a person doesn't have his word, then he doesn't have anything. It so so true. How do you know if a chiropractor is honest when you first visit their office? That's a hard one to answer. It may simply be a "gut" sort of thing. But usually, if we trust our "gut", then we don't get steered off of the right track.

You may not be able to develop a "gut" feeling until the second or third visit but you will most likely get a good idea by then. I would say that, in general, if the exam consists of simply 'bouncing' up and down the spine with the fingers, finding several sore spots, and then making them make popping noises, then you are not in a good place and need to leave. For a good, solid exam and evaluation, the first visit is typically going to last thirty minutes to an hour. Minimum.

In addition, if it takes 3 visits to get your recommendations and really start treating, they may be using sales tactics on you.

If they talk about having to see them once a week for a year or for a lifetime, they may not necessarily be dishonest but they are most certainly unaware of current guidelines and evidence-based protocols.

If they talk about fixing everything in your body based on a subluxation model, I'd say you should save your money and leave. That's just me. Again, that doesn't mean dishonesty but it does mean they may not be evidence-based because the evidence and research cannot back that sort of treatment.

If x-rays are taken of you on the first visit and big ordeal is made of the lack of curvature in your neck and you are offered 35, 45, even 75 visits over the course of a year to get it fixed, just understand that there are several high-level, longitudinal studies (mentioned in this book) that do not support that sort of treatment.

If you are offered a contract for treatment, it is my opinion that you turn around and run out. Don't walk.

There is a group of younger chiropractors out there in the world convincing their patients that they can remove degenerative spinal bone spurs through adjustments 2-3 times per day for 3 weeks. Again, research I am aware of does not support this and neither should anyone else.

EVIDENCE-BASED/EVIDENCE INFORMED

OK, this one is admittedly a sticky one here. As most chiropractors are well-aware, there is a huge chasm in our profession between those that believe in only adjusting the spine and nothing else and those that are evidence-based or evidence-informed.

Between those that follow a philosophy and those that follow research. Between those that do not believe in the profession progressing and growing and those that believe our profession can and should grow and expand.

There are some research papers that the philosophy group will point to saying these papers prove their theories and minimal treatment but, in truth, from what I've seen, they are low quality and no profession worth anything would rest their entire reputation on them.

However, there are **TONS** of papers, many of which we have covered on the Chiropractic Forward Podcast, and here in this book, that prove and validate evidence-based chiropractic every day in almost every way.

In general, it is my recommendation that you **BE** the chiropractor or refer your family **TO** the chiropractor that follows research, follows the expanding knowledge within, and pushes to move the profession more and more into the current century.

NETWORK

To me, "Network" means, "how plugged in is the doctor as far as his associations, his colleagues, and the profession as a whole?"

On the surface, that may sound like a silly suggestion and to be somewhat inconsequential to anything. But I have found that there is an extreme amount of value in being active with fellow chiropractors and state and national associations.

We are able to bounce ideas and questions off of each other whereas someone with no colleague interaction or support system merely has their own knowledge, dogma, bias, and ideology and is sort of on an island of their own making.

Trust me, this is coming from a practitioner that was on that self-made island years and years ago. I had my basic knowledge from going to chiropractic school but I wasn't particularly skilled in anything extra.

Just basic white paint in a world of oranges, purple, lilac, or whatever color you can think of. Sitting here today, I wouldn't send anyone to me back then if I am being honest.

Being active and involved in the Texas Chiropractic Association has allowed me the opportunity to stay plugged in with rules and regulations, new treatments, changes in insurance plans, and options that I would have likely never known about were I not being active in my profession and well-networked with my colleagues.

KNOWLEDGE & EXPERIENCE OF DOCTOR AND STAFF

I think this qualification really goes without saying. And again, knowledge and experience is of extreme importance in ANY profession. Even an experienced comedian is usually going put on a better show than a rookie.

For instance, I attend a chiropractic conference one weekend out of every month. Chiropractors are required 16 hours of continuing education every year. Some chiropractors will only go to a continuing education seminar one weekend out of every year. I should know, I used to be one of those chiropractors. Let's be honest here, many see this as a weekend out of town and look for every way possible to skip those hours and have a fun weekend while still getting their 'hours' in.

But with age comes wisdom and the desire for more wisdom. I would do my best to figure out the chiropractor's knowledge and their level of experience. This could certainly end up being a "gut" thing as we previously discussed but it's usually something they are proud of and something they proudly display and market. I know I do. There should be nobody in my local area that is not aware by now that I have a Fellowship or that I am certified in Whiplash Biomechanics & Traumatology. I earned it and the only way it makes me any return on investment is if I effectively tell others about it.

If there's no sign on the website of extra certification and achievement, your money is probably best spent elsewhere. I'm ten times the doctor I was when I began the Diplomate program. Or more....exponentially better.

GOOD LISTENER

You are not going to be able to get this off of a doctor's website so don't even try but we can strive to be better ourselves in this department. Myself included. I have been at a point where I did not feel I could get everyone worked through in one day and I can guarantee you I cut some patients off in the middle of their explanation.

I think that it is very important that a doctor has a good bedside manner. Meaning, that they need to be able to listen, focus on the patient, and fully understand what the patient is saying and what their concerns are. There are those days where we are just doing everything we can to stay above water but in general, don't be uninterested and think you have the problem solved before they've said anything.

As Dr. Stuart McGill has suggested, for many patients, they have just never had someone listen to their story. He begins his evaluation by sitting in chairs across from each other and simply asking the patient to tell their story. That sounds like a good start to being a good listener.

Open your ears.

OFFICE PRESENTATION.

This may seem like a silly one and I'm sorry if it is just not important to you, but if I am going to a doctor's office, I expect the office to be mostly clean and fairly sharp looking.

I think that if a healthcare provider takes pride in their office space and in their staff, then they are going to take pride in their results and their expertise. You can find those that do not give a squat about anything in their office. No nice pictures or decor, old this, smelly that..yet they're able to get the best results.

Let's face it though, is that the exception or the rule? I argue it's the exception.

In what I think is an ideal office, they try to have a welcoming feeling, the staff is dressed neatly, there is as little dirt or dust is on the floor and furniture as is possible, there is no trash on the floor next to the trash can, everything is as nice, as sharp, and as clean as possible.

It is the Disney concept of 'front of stage' and 'back of stage'. Everything the audience (your patients) sees should be sharp, clean, appealing, and professional.

If the doctor and the staff do not portray an acceptable image, then that may not be the place for you.

A SENSE OF PURPOSE

Have you ever gone to a doctor's office and felt that they were simply going through the motions and collecting money? Crackin' necks and cashin' checks!!

I have absolutely felt that way a time or two. I think that the better doctor is genuinely concerned about his patients' well-being, and how he can help them in the best way possible.

Someone that you can just feel is a little extra. Someone that is knowledgeable and can relate things to you in understandable terms. Not chiropractic jargon. Someone that you can instantly tell is not there to get into your pocket or to max your insurance. Someone that does not treat you like a sales target that is to be 'closed' for as many visits and dollars as possible.

You know what I'm talking about. Someone that is there to get you results as quickly as possible.

That's purpose.

Even on top of that though, it would be nice to find a chiropractor that you felt had the community's best interest in mind. When you see them donating and giving back to their community, why wouldn't you want to do business with that person instead of a taker.

Takers just take. They never give back or put back in. Takers just make profit but are narcissistic. They don't get involved with their state or national associations at all. They don't give anything back to their profession, their school, or their community.

They take that money and spend it only on themselves because that's all they care about. I don't want to do business with that person. I want to do business with a giver. Any day all day. Gimme a giver.

Thank you, i'll have another please.

I want a chiropractor that got into the profession of chiropractic in order to heal people. And to heal as many people as he could possibly reach. Not to 'close' them and treat them like cattle. Someone that thinks and works on a higher level rather than someone that just shows up to work and does their job. A doctor that is excited and jazzed to be doing what they're doing in the place where they are doing it.

THAT'S the practitioner I want to go to!

KNOWS WHEN TO REFER

When we talk about referrals, we can get way off track in the chiropractic profession. Some chiropractors feel they can solve any problem walking through their doors. Ear infection? Pop ya bones! Asthma? Pop ya bones. Cancer? Pop ya bones. Diverticulitis? Pop ya bones! Bad lunch? Pop ya bones!

They're the reason people in the medical field look at all of us like we're crazy. And if that's the measuring stick for crazy, then they're right. Fortunately, most of us aren't like that. But the loud minority is still winning the day in our profession when it comes to this sort of behavior, I'm afraid.

The recent COVID-19 pandemic was the perfect evidence of a profession at odds with itself. When you have so many up in arms over vaccinations, mask-wearing, and protective measures because they assert that weekly adjustments by a chiropractor boosts the immune system enough to protect their patients form COVID, well, that is all you need to see to realize there is still a big problem. A big problem with chiropractors not understanding research literature or even knowing about the literature. A big problem with those chiropractors not understanding what is or is not within their capabilities. Or what is or is not within their scope of practice.

As I said before, I am interested in the chiropractor that is plugged in to his profession and to his colleagues. I'm interested in the chiropractor that is plugged in to the healthcare field as a whole. And I'm absolutely interested in the chiropractor who is plugged into research and current, accepted guidelines. For a so-called healthcare profession that wishes to survive well into the future, I see no other way to proceed.

If a doctor gives me a sense that they feel that they are the only one that can handle any condition, or that there is never any need to look outside of their office for additional help, then I am likely going to find another doctor. I think it is extremely important to go to a doctor that is not afraid to admit when additional treatment should be reasonably looked at.

I for one, look forward to each and every time that I have the opportunity to work in conjunction with a medical provider. I feel that it is a very complete treatment plan when you are able to address all symptoms thoroughly.

Patients have to take into consideration whether they want a chiropractor that is deeply versed in chiropractic philosophy or want a chiropractor that is on top of current, high-level research and is open to working with the medical community.

LOVE.

I like to throw curveballs here and there. I like to add things you don't see in most lists. This is one of those things and I saved this one for last because I hope that, after you are done reading this, this is the one that will resonate the longest with you.

I strongly feel that when you visit a health care provider, things like caring, genuineness, focus, listening, and all of those other things that we've talked about above.....they can all be wrapped up into one thing.

And I think that that one thing is 'LOVE'. If the doctor and the staff love what they do, they love their patients, and they love being where they are, when they are there, then people can feel that.

If you walk into an office and it's cold, there's no personality, and it feels stiff and stale, then that's just no fun at all. Where's the love?

How do you show it to your patients? Think about it.

I want an office that I love to go to and if the doctor and the staff have love as the primary driver of their office and their purpose and it's something palpable that you can feel, then I think all of the other eight characteristics pretty much take care of themselves.

So, proceed with love.

Jeff S. Williams, DC, FIANM

URGENT PLEA!

THANK YOU FOR READING MY BOOK!

I truly appreciate all of your feedback and thoughts with regard to this book. I love hearing what you have to say.

I need your input so that I can make sure the next version of this book and future books are as good as they can possibly be.

Please leave me a helpful review on Amazon letting me know what you thought of the book. It would be so helpful!

Thank you so much and God Bless.

- Jeff Williams, DC, FIANM

BIBLIOGRAPHY

1. *Introduction To Evidence-Based Practice.* Sep 21, 2016 1:42 AM; Available from: http://guides.mclibrary.duke.edu/c. php?g=158201&p=1036068.
2. *Professional Comparison.* Available from: https://prohealthsys.com/students/professional-comparison/.
3. Sandefur R, e.a., "Assessment of knowledge of primary care activities in a sample of medical and chiropractic students.". J Manipulative Physiol Ther, Jun 2005. **28**(5): p. 336-44.
4. Taylor JA, e.a., Interpretation of abnormal lumbosacral spine radiographs. A test comparing students, clinicians, radiology residents, and radiologists in medicine and chiropractic. Spine (Phila Pa 1976), 1995. **20**(10): p. 1147-53.
5. Matzkin E, e.a., Adequacy of education in musculoskeletal medicine. J Bone Joint Surg Am, 2005 Feb. **87**(2): p. 310-4.
6. Goncalves G, L.S., Leboeuf-Yde,, Effect of chiropractic treatment on primary or early secondary prevention: a systematic review with a pedagogic approach. Chiropr Man Therap, 2018.
7. Goertz C, Adding chiropractic manipulative therapy to standard medical care for patients with acute low back pain: Results from a pragmatic randomized comparative effectiveness study. Spine, 2013. **38**(8): p. 627-634.
8. Muller R, G.L., Long-term follow-up of a randomized clinical trial assessing the efficacy of medication, acupuncture, and spinal manipulation for chronic mechanical spinal pain syndromes. J Manipulative Physiol Ther., 2005. **28**(1): p. 3-11.
9. Meade TW, D.S., Browne W, et. al., Low back pain of mechanical origin: randomized comparison of chiropractic and hospital outpatient treatment. Br Med J, 1990. **300**: p. 1431-1437.
10. Herzog W, e.a., Electromyographic responses of back and limb muscles associated with spinal manipulative therapy. Spine (Phila Pa 1976), 1999. **24**(2): p. 146-52.
11. Senna MK, Does maintained spinal manipulation therapy for chronic nonspecific low back pain result in better long-term outcome? Spine (Phila Pa 1976), 2011. **Aug 15; 36**(18): p. 1427-37.

Jeff S. Williams, DC, FIANM

12. Hill JC, W.D., Lewis M,, Comparison of stratified primary care management for low back pain with current best practice (STarTBack): a randomised controlled trial. Lancet, 2011. **378**: p. 1560-71.
13. Wiegel PA, e.a., Chiropractic us in teh medicare population: prevalence, patterns, and associations with 1-year changes in health and satisfaction with care. J Manipulative Physiol Ther, 2014. **37**(8): p. 542-51.
14. Axen I, H.L., Leboeuf-Yde C,, Chiropractic maintenance care - what's new? A systematic review of the literature. Chiropr Man Therap, 2019. **27**(63).
15. Eklund A, The Nordic Maintenance Care program: Effectiveness of chiropractic maintenance care versus symptom-guided treatment for recurrent and persistent low back pain—A pragmatic randomized controlled trial. PLoS One, 2018. **13**(9).
16. Eklund A, J.I., Leboeuf-Yde C, Kongsted A, Jonsson M, Lovgren P,, The Nordic Maintenance Care Program: Does psychological profile modify the treatment effect of a preventive manual therapy intervention? A secondary analysis of a pragmatic randomized controlled trial. PLoS One, 2019.
17. Eklund A, HJ., Jensen I, Leboeuf-Yde C,, The Nordic maintenance care program: maintenance care reduces the number of days with pain in acute episodes and increases the length of pain free periods for dysfunctional patients with recurrent and persistent low back pain - a secondary analysis of a pragmatic randomized controlled trial. Chiropr Man Therap, 2020. **28**(19).
18. Sarnat R, e.a., Clinical and Cost Outcomes of an Integrative Medicine IPA. J Manipulative Physiol Ther, 2004. **27**(5): p. 336-347.
19. Enke O, Anticonvulsants in the treatment of low back pain and lumbar radicular pain: a systematic review and meta-analysis. CMAJ, 2018(190): p. E786-93.
20. Underwood M, United Kingdom back pain exercise and manipulation (UK BEAM) randomised trial: effectiveness of physical treatments for back pain in primary care: UK BEAM Trial. BMJ, 2004. **329**(7479): p. 1377.
21. Manga P, e.a., THE MANGA REPORT: THE EFFECTIVENESS AND COST-EFFECTIVENESS OF CHIROPRACTIC MANAGEMENT OF LOW BACK-PAIN. Funded by the Ontario Ministry of Health, 1993.

22. Vickers AJ, V.E., Lewith G., Acupuncture for Chronic Pain: Update of an Individual Patient Data Meta-Analysis. J Pain, 2018. **19**(5): p. 455-474.

23. Meade TW, D.S., Browne W, Frank AO, Randomized comparison of chiropractic and hospital outpatient management for low back pain: Results from extended follow up. Br Med J, 1995. **311**(7001): p. 349-351.

24. Sussman B, Wellness-related Use Of Common Complementary Health Approaches Among Adults: The United States, 2012. National Health Statistics Reports, 2015. **85**.

25. Tsertsvadze A, e.a., Cost-effectiveness of manual therapy for the management of musculoskeletal conditions: a systematic review and narrative synthesis of evidence from randomized controlled trials. J Manipulative Physiol Ther, 2014. **37**(6): p. 343-62.

26. Giles LGF, M.R., Chronic spinal pain syndromes: a clinical pilot trial comparing acupuncture, a nonsteroidal anti-inflammatory drug, and spinal manipulation. J Manipulative Physiol Ther, 1999. **22**(6): p. 376-81.

27. Korthals-de Bos IB, Cost effectiveness of physiotherapy, manual therapy, and general practitioner care for neck pain: economic evaluation alongside a randomised controlled trial. British Medical Journal, 2003. **326**(7395): p. 911.

28. Peterson CK, Symptomatic, Magnetic Resonance Imaging-Confirmed Cervical Disk Herniation Patients: A Comparative-Effectiveness Prospective Observational Study of 2 Age- and Sex-Matched Cohorts Treated With Either Imaging-Guided Indirect Cervical Nerve Root Injections or Spinal Manipulative Therapy. J Manipulative Physiol Ther, 2016. **39**(3): p. 210-7.

29. Taco AW, e.a., First-Contact Care With a Medical vs Chiropractic Provider After Consultation With a Swiss Telemedicine Provider: Comparison of Outcomes, Patient Satisfaction, and Health Care Costs in Spinal, Hip, and Shoulder Pain Patients. J Manipulative Physiol Ther, 2015. **38**(7): p. 477-483.

30. Bronfort G, Efficacy of spinal manipulation for chronic headache: a systematic review. J Manipulative Physiol Ther, 2001. **24**(7): p. 457-466.

31. Li L, e.a., Systematic review of clinical randomized controlled trials on manipulative treatment of lumbar disc herniation. Zhongguo Gu Shang, 2010. **23**(9): p. 696-700.

32. Chou R, Epidural Corticosteroid Injections for Radiculopathy and Spinal Stenosis: A Systematic Review and Meta-analysis. Ann Intern Med, 2015. **163**(5): p. 373-81.

33. Bronfort G, Efficacy of spinal manipulation and mobilization for low back pain and neck pain: a systematic review and best evidence synthesis. Spine, 2004. **May-Jun 4**(3): p. 335-56.

34. Hurwitz EL, e.a., Variations in Patterns of Utilization and Charges for the Care of Neck Pain in North Carolina, 2000 to 2009: A Statewide Claims' Data Analysis. J Manipulative Physiol Ther, 2016. **May 39**(4): p. 240-51.

35. Whedon JM, e.a., Risk of traumatic injury associated with chiropractic spinal manipulation in Medicare Part B beneficiaries aged 66 to 99 years. Spine (Phila Pa 1976), 2015. **40**(4): p. 264-270.

36. Nelson CF, e.a., The efficacy of spinal manipulation, amitriptyline and the combination of both therapies for prophylaxis of migraine headache. Journal of Manipulative and Physiological Therapeutics, 1998. **Oct 21**(8): p. 511-19.

37. 3Deyo RA, Overtreating chronic back pain: time to back off? J Am Board Fam Med, 2009. **22**(1): p. 62-8.

38. Haas M, A practice-based study of patients with acute and chronic low back pain attending primary care and chiropractic physicians: two-week to 48-month follow-up. J Manipulative Physiol Ther, 2004. **Mar-Apr;27**(3): p. 160-9.

39. Chou R, Surgery for low back pain: a review of the evidence for an American Pain Society Clinical Practice Guideline. Spine, 2009. **34**(10): p. 1094-109.

40. Keeney BJ, Early predictors of lumbar spine surgery after occupational back injury: results from a prospective study of workers in Washington State. Spine (Phila Pa 1976), 2013. **May 15**(38): p. 11.

41. Martins DE, e.a., Quality assessment of systematic reviews for surgical treatment of low back pain: an overview. Spine J, 2016. **16**(5): p. 667-75.

42. Maghout J, e.e., Lumbar fusion outcomes in Washington State workers' compensation. Spine (Phila Pa 1976), 2006. **31**(23): p. 2715-23.

43. Chou R, e.a., Diagnosis and Treatment of Low Back Pain: A Joint Clinical Practice Guideline from the American College of Physicians and the American Pain Society. Ann Intern Med, 2007. **147**(7): p. 478-91.

44. Schneider M, Comparison of spinal manipulation methods and usual medical care for acute and subacute low back pain: a randomized clinical trial. Spine, 2015. **Feb 15; 40**(4): p. 209-217.

45. Nyiendo J, Pain, disability, and satisfaction outcomes and predictors of outcomes: A practice-based study of chronic low back pain patients attending primary care and chiropractic physicians. J Manipulative Physiol Ther, 2001. **24**(7): p. 433-39.

46. Kuligowski R, D.-B.A., Skrzek A,, Effectiveness of Traction in Young Patients Representing Different Stages of Degenerative Disc Disease. J Orthop Tramuatol Rehabil, 2019. **21**(3): p. 187-195.

47. Licciardone J, Osteopathic manipulative treatment for low back pain: a systematic review and meta-analysis of randomized controlled trials. BMC Musculoskeletal Disorders, 2005. **43**(6).

48. Lawrence, D., Chiropractic management of low back pain and low back-related leg complaints: a literature synthesis. J Manipulative Physiol Ther, Nove-Dec. 2008.

49. Reports, C. Relief for aching backs *Hands-on therapies were top-reated by 14,000 consumers.* 2009; Available from: http://www.consumerreports.org/cro/magazine-archive/may-2009/health/back-pain/overview/back-pain-ov.htm?rurl=http%3A%2F%2Fwww.consumerreports.org%2Fcro%2Fmagazine-archive%2Fmay-2009%2Fhealth%2Fback-pain%2Foverview%2Fback-pain-ov.htm%3FloginMethod%3Dauto.

50. Vieira-Pellenz F, e.a., Short-term effect of spinal manipulation on pain perception, spinal mobility, and full height recovery in male subjects with degenerative disk disease: a randomized controlled trial. *Randomized controlled trial.* Arch Phys Med Rehabil, 2014. **95**(9): p. 1613-9.

51. Bishop P, The C.H.I.R.O. (Chiropractic Hospital-Based Interventions Research Outcomes) Study. Dynamic Chiropractic Canada, 2008. **8**(11).

52. Hidalgo B, The efficacy of manual therapy and exercise for different stages of non-specific low back pain: an update of systematic reviews. J Man Manip Ther, 2014. **May 22**(2): p. 59-74.

53. Wolfgang J, e.a., Spinal HVLA-Manipulation in Acute Nonspecific LBP: A Double Blinded Randomized Controlled Trial in Comparison With Diclofenac and Placebo. Spine, 2012. **38**(7).

54. Choi B, e.a., Exercises for prevention of recurrences of low-back pain. The Cochrane database of systematic reviews, 2010.

55. Hertzman-Miller R, e.a., Comparing the Satisfaction of Low Back Pain Patients Randomized to Receive Medical or Chiropractic Care: Results From the UCLA Low-Back Pain Study. Am J Public Health, 2002. **92**(10): p. 1628-1633.
56. Troyanovich SJ, H.D., Harrison DE, Low back pain and the lumbar intervertebral disk: Clinical consideration for the doctor of chiropractic. Journal of Manipulative and Physiological Therapeutics, 1999. **22**(2): p. 96-104.
57. Leemann S, Outcome of acute and chronic patients with magnetic resonance imaging-confirmed symptomatic lumbar disc herniations receiving high-velocity, lo-amplitude, spinal manipulative therapy: a prospective observational cohort study with one-year follow-up. J Manipulative Physiol Ther, 2014. **Mar-Apr 37**(3): p. 155-163.
58. Visser LH, e.a., Treatment of the sacroiliac joint in patients with leg pain: a randomized-controlled trial. Eur Spine J, 2013. **22**(10): p. 2310-7.
59. Kamali F, e.a., The effect of two manipulative therapy techniques and their outcome in patients with sacroiliac joint syndrome. J Bodyw Mov Ther, 2012. **16**(1).
60. La Touche R, G.S., Garcia B,, Effect of Manual Therapy and Therapeutic Exercise Applied to the Cervical Region on Pain and Pressure Pain Sensitivity in Patients with Temporomandibular Disorders: A Systematic Review and Meta-analysis. Pain Med, 2020.
61. Bronfort G, Effectiveness of manual therapies: The UK evidence report. Chiropr Osteopat, 2010. **18**(3).
62. Saayman L, e.a., Chiropractic manipulative therapy and low-level laser therapy in the management of cervical facet dysfunction: a randomized controlled study. J Manipulative Physiol Ther, 2011. **34**(3): p. 153-63.
63. Evans R, Two-year follow-up of a randomized clinical trial of spinal manipulation and two types of exercise for patients with chronic neck pain. Spine (Phila Pa 1976), 2002. **27**(21): p. 2383-9.
64. Chaibi A, R.M., A risk-benefit assessment strategy to exclude cervical artery dissection in spinal manual-therapy: A comprehensive review. Annals of Medicine, 2018.
65. Guzman J, Clinical Practice Implications of the Bone and Joint Decade 2000–2010 Task Force on Neck Pain and Its Associated Disorders: From Concepts and Findings to Recommendations. Spine, 2008. **33**(4S): p. S199-S213.

66. Dagenais S. Summary review of the scieentific evidence on the harms and efficacy of commonly used therapies for neck pain, including manual therapies, therapeutic exercises, and medication. Available from: http://www.acatoday.org/pdf/NeckPainTreatments.pdf.

67. Cassidy, e.a., Risk of Vertebrobasilar Stroke and Chiropractic Car. Spine, 2008. **33**(4S): p. S176-S183.

68. June 29-30, 2009: Joint Meeting of the Drug Safety and Risk Management Advisory Committee with the Anesthetic and Life Support Drugs Advisory Committee and the Nonprescription Drugs Advisory Committee: Meeting Announcement. 2013; Available from: http://www.fda.gov/AdvisoryCommittees/Calendar/ucm143083.htm.

69. Wolfe MM, Gastrointestinal toxicity of nonsteroidal anti-inflammatory drugs. NEJM, 1999. **340**: p. 1888.

70. Bhala N, e.a., Vascular and upper gastrointestinal effects of non-steroidal anti-inflammatory drugs: meta-analyses of individual participant data from randomised trials. Lancet, 2013. **382**(9894): p. 769-79.

71. *Data sheet for VALIUM® brand of diazepam tablets.*; Available from: http://www.accessdata.fda.gov/drugsatfda_docs/label/2008/013263s083lbl.pdf.

72. Jones CM, e.a., Pharmaceutical Overdose Deaths, Unites States, 2010. JAMA, 2013. **309**(7): p. 657-59.

73. Bronfort G, Spinal Manipulation, Medication, or Home Exercise With Advice for Acute and Subacute Neck Pain: A Randomized Trial. Annals of Internal Medicine 2012. Ann Intern Med, 2012. **156**(1): p. 1-10.

74. Herzog W, e.a., Vertebral artery strains during high-speed, low amplitude cervical spinal manipulation. J Electromyography and Kenisiology, 2012. **22**(5): p. 740-746.

75. Debette S, "Pathophysiology and risk factors of cervical artery dissection: what have we learnt from large hospital-based cohorts?". Current Opinion in Neurology, 2014. **27**(1): p. 20-8.

76. Lang E. *Vertebral Artery Dissection.* Emergency Medicine 2017 January 18]; Available from: https://emedicine.medscape.com/article/761451-overview.

77. Mutikani L. *Opioid crisis cost U.S. economy $504 billion in 2015: White House.* 2017; Available from: https://www.reuters.com/article/legal-us-usa-opioids-cost/opioid-crisis-cost-u-s-economy-504-billion-in-2015-white-house-idUSKBN1DL2Q0.

Jeff S. Williams, DC, FIANM

78. Glenza J. *Life expectancy in US down for second year in a row as opioid crisis deepens.* 2017 December 21; Available from: https://www.theguardian.com/us-news/2017/dec/21/us-life-expectancy-down-for-second-year-in-a-row-amid-opioid-crisis.

79. Epstein N, The risks of epidural and transforaminal steroid injections in the Spine: Commentary and a comprehensive review of the literature. Surg Neurol Int, 2013. **4**(Suppl 2): p. S74-93.

80. Dewitte V, Articular dysfunction patterns in patients with mechanical neck pain: a clinical algorithm to guide specific mobilization and manipulation techniques. Man Ther, 2014. **19**(2-9).

81. Dunning J, Upper cervical and upper thoracic manipulation versus mobilization and exercise in patients with cervicogenic headache: a multi-center randomized clinical trial. BMC Musculoskeletal Disorders, 2016. **16**(64).

82. Yu H, Upper cervical manipulation combined with mobilization for the treatment of atlantoaxial osteoarthritis: a report of 10 cases. J Manipulative Physiol Ther, 2011. **34**(2): p. 131-7.

83. Puentedura EJ, Thoracic spine thrust manipulation versus cervical spine thrust manipulation in patients with acute neck pain: a randomized clinical trial. J Orthop Sports Phys Ther, 2011. **41**(4): p. 208-20.

84. Tuchin PJ, e.a., A randomized controlled trial of chiropractic spinal manipulative therapy for migraine. J Manipulative Physiol Ther, 2000. **23**(2): p. 91-95.

85. McCrory D, Behavioral and Physical Treatments for Tension-type and Cervicogenic Headache. Duke University Evidence-based Practice Center, Center for Clinical Health Policy Research.

86. Kosloff T, e.a., Chiropractic care and the risk of vertebrobasilar stroke: results of a case–control study in U.S. commercial and Medicare Advantage populations. Chiropractic & Manual Therapies, 2015. **23**(19).

87. Quesnele JJ, e.a., Changes in vertebral artery blood flow following various head positions and cervical spine manipulation. J Manipulative Physiol Ther, 2014. **37**(1): p. 22-31.

88. Buzzatti L, e.a., Atlanto-axial facet displacement during rotational high-velocity low-amplitude thrust: An in vitro 3D kinematic analysis. Man Ther, 2015. **20**(6): p. 783-9.

89. Achalandabaso A, e.a., Tissue damage markers after a spinal manipulation in healthy subjects: a preliminary report of a randomized controlled trial. Dis Markers, 2014.

90. Church E, e.a., Systematic Review and Meta-analysis of Chiropractic Care and Cervical Artery Dissection: No Evidence for Causation. Cureus, 2016. **8**(2): p. e498.

91. Okada E, D.K., Fujiwara H, Nishiwaki Y,, Twenty-year Longitudinal Follow-up MRI Study of Asymptomatic Volunteers: The Impact of Cervical Alignment on Disk Degeneration. Clin Spine Surg, 2018. **31**(10): p. 446-451.

92. Daimon K, F.H., Nishiwaki Y,, A 20-year prospective longitudinal MRI study on cervical spine after whiplash injury: Follow-up of a cross-sectional study. J Ortho Science, 2019. **24**(4): p. 579-583.

93. Lippa L, L.L., Cacciola F,, Loss of cervical lordosis: What is the prognosis? J Craniovertebr Junction Spine, 2017. **8**(1): p. 9-14.

94. Guo G, L.J., Diao Q,, Cervical lordosis in asymptomatic individuals: a meta-analysis. J Orthop Surg Res, 2018. **13**(147).

95. Goncalves G, D.M., Leboeuf-Yde C, Wedderkopp N,, Chiropractic conservatism and the ability to determine contra-indications, non-indications, and indications to chiropractic care: a cross-sectional survey of chiropractic students. BMC Chiro Man Ther, 2019. **27**(3).

96. Espi-Lopez G, e.a., Do manual therapy techniques have a positive effect on quality of life in people with tension-type headache? A randomized controlled trial. Eur J Phys Rehabil Med, 2016. **13**(1): p. 4-13.

97. Fritz J, e.a., Preliminary investigation of the mechanisms underlying the effects of manipulation: exploration of a multi-variate model including spinal stiffness, multifidus recruitment, and clinical findings. Spine (Phila Pa 1976), 2011. **36**(21): p. 1772-1781.

98. Aure OF, e.a., Manual therapy and exercise therapy in patients with chronic low back pain: A randomized, controlled trial with 1-year follow-up. Spine, 2003. **28**(6): p. 525-532.

99. Nguyen HS, e.a., Upright magnetic resonance imaging of the lumbar spine: Back pain and radiculopathy. J Craniovertebr Junction Spine, 2016. **7**(1): p. 31-7.

100. Madsen R, e.a., The effect of body position and axial load on spinal canal morphology: an MRI study of central spinal stenosis. Spine (Phila Pa 1976), 2008. **33**(1): p. 61-7.

Jeff S. Williams, DC, FIANM

101. Hansson T, e.a., The narrowing of the lumbar spinal canal during loaded MRI: the effects of the disc and ligamentum flavum. Eur Spine J, 2009. **18**(5): p. 679-86.

102. Choy DS, Magnetic resonance imaging of the lumbosacral spine under compression. J Clin Laseer Med Surg, 1997. **15**(2): p. 71-3.

103. Nowicki BH, e.a., Occult lumbar lateral spinal stenosis in neural foramina subjected to physiologic loading. AJNR Am J Neuroraiol, 1996. **17**(9): p. 1605-14.

104. Willen J, e.a., The diagnostic effect from axial loading of the lumbar spine during computed tomography and magnetic resonance imaging in patients with degenerative disorders. Spine (Phila Pa 1976), 2001. **26**(23): p. 2607-14.

105. Ferreiro P, e.a., Evaluation of intervertebral disc herniation and hypermobile intersegmental instability in symptomatic adult patients undergoing recumbent and upright MRI of the cervical or lumbosacral spines. Eur J Radiol, 2007. **62**(3): p. 444-8.

106. Ahn TJ, e.a., Effect of intervertebral disk degeneration on spinal stenosis during magnetic resonance imaging with axial loading. Neurol Med Chir (Tokyo), 2009. **49**(6): p. 242-7.

107. Willen J, e.a., Dynamic effects on the lumbar spinal canal: axially loaded CT-myelography and MRI in patients with sciatica and/or neurogenic claudication. Spine (Phila Pa 1976), 1997. **22**(24): p. 2968-76.

108. Kanno H, e.a., Axial loading during magnetic resonance imaging in patients with lumbar spinal canal stenosis: does it reproduce the positional change of the dural sac detected by upright myelography? Spine (Phila Pa 1976), 2012. **37**(16): p. E985-92.

109. Danielson B, e.a., Axially loaded magnetic resonance image of the lumbar spine in asymptomatic individuals. Spine (Phila Pa 1976), 2001. **26**(23): p. 2601-6.

110. Benson RT, Conservatively treated massive prolapsed discs: a 7-year follow-up. Ann R Coll Surg, 2010. **92**(2): p. 147-153.

111. Peterson C, e.a., Outcomes from magnetic resonance imaging – confirmed symptomatic cervical disk protrusion patients treated with high-velocity, low-amplitude spinal manipulative therapy: a prospective cohort study with 3-month follow-up. J Manipulative Physiol Ther, 2013. **36**(8): p. 461-7.

112. Eyerman E, e.a., MRI Evidence of Nonsurgical, Mechanical Reduction, Rehydration and Repair of the herniated Lumbar Disc. J Neuro Imaging, 1998. **8**(2).

113. Apfel CC, e.a., Restoration of disk height through non-surgical spinal decompression is associated with decreased discogenic low back pain: a retrospective cohort study. BMC Musculoskelet Disord, 2010. **11**: p. 155.

114. Shealy N, e.a., Emerging Technologies: Preliminary Findings: DECOMPRESSION, REDUCTION, AND STABILIZATION OF THE LUMBAR SPINE: A COST-EFFECTIVE TREATMENT FOR LUMBOSACRAL PAIN. Am J Pain Management, 1997. **7**(2).

115. Kuo YW, e.a., Spinal traction promotes molecular transportation in a simulated degenerative intervertebral disc model. Spine (Phila Pa 1976), 2014. **39**(9): p. E550-6.

116. Qaseem A, Noninvasive Treatments for Acute, Subacute, and Chronic Low Back Pain: A Clinical Practice Guideline From the American College of Physicians. Ann Intern Med, 2017. **4**(166): p. 514-530.

117. Chen YJ, e.a., Effect of low level laser therapy on chronic compression of the dorsal root ganglion. PLoS One, 2014. **9**(3).

118. Alghadir A, e.a., Effect of low-level laser therapy in patients with chronic knee osteoarthritis: a single-blinded randomized clinical study. Lasers Med Sci, 2014. **29**(2): p. 749-55.

119. Gasperini G, Does low-level laser therapy decrease swelling and pain resulting from orthognathic surgery? Int J Oral Maxillofac Surg, 2014. **43**(7): p. 868-73.

120. ZeYu H, e.a., The effectiveness of low-level laser therapy for nonspecific chronic low back pain: a systematic review and meta-analysis. Arthritis Research & Therapy, 2015. **17**.

121. Soleimanpour H, e.a., The effect of low-level laser therapy on knee osteoarthritis: prospective, descriptive study. Lasers Med Sci, 2014. **29**(5): p. 1695-700.

122. Pereira TS, e.a., Efficacy of red and infrared lasers in treatment of temporomandibular disorders--a double-blind, randomized, parallel clinical trial. Cranio, 2014. **32**(1): p. 51-6.

123. George JW, e.a., A randomized controlled trial comparing a multimodal intervention and standard obstetrics care for low back and pelvic pain in pregnancy. Am J Obstet Gynecol., 2013. **208**(4): p. 295.

124. Peterson C, e.a., Outcomes of pregnant patients with low back pain undergoing chiropractic treatment: a prospective cohort study with short term, medium term, and 1 year follow-up. Chiropr Man Therap, 2014. **22**(1): p. 15.

125. Majchrzycki M, e.a., Application of osteopathic manipulative technique in the treatment of back pain during pregnancy. Genkol Pol, 2015. **86**(3): p. 224-8.

126. Bernard M, Chiropractic Management of Pregnancy-Related Lumbopelvic Pain: A Case Study. J Chiropr Med, 2016. **15**(2): p. 129-33.

127. Lisi AJ, Chiropractic spinal manipulation for low back pain of pregnancy: a retrospective case series. J Midwifery Womens Health, 2006. **51**(1): p. e7-10.

128. Sadr S, e.a., The treatment experience of patients with low back pain during pregnancy and their chiropractors: a qualitative study. Chiropr Man Therap, 2012. **20**(1): p. 32.

129. Khan S, e.a., Asymptomatic classification of whiplash injury and the implications for treatment. Journal of Orthopaedic Medicine, 1999. **21**(1): p. 22-25.

130. Nolet PS, N.L., Kristman VL, Croft AC, Zeegers MP, Freeman MD,, Is Acceleration a Valid Proxy for Injury Risk in Minimal Damage Traffic Crashes? A Comparative Review of Volunteer, ADL and Real-World Studies. Int J Environ Res Public Health, 2021. **18**(6): p. 2901.

131. Freeman MD, L.W., Estimating the number of traffic crash-related cervical spine injuries in the United States; An analysis and comparison of national crash and hospital data. Accid Anal Prev, 2020. **142**(105571).

132. Fernandez-de-las-Penas C, F.-C.J., Palomeque del Cerro L, Miangolarra-Page JC, Manipulative treatment vs. conventional physiotherapy treatment in whiplash injury: a randomized controlled trial. J Whip Rel Dis, 2004. **3**: p. 73-90.

133. Williamson E, e.a., Risk factors for chronic disability in a cohort of patients with acute whiplash associated disorders seeking physiotherapy treatment for persisting symptoms. Physiotherapy, 2015. **101**(1): p. 34-43.

134. Borchgrevink GE, e.a., National health insurance consumption and chronic symptoms following mild neck sprain injuries in car collisions. Scand J Soc Med, 1996. **24**(4): p. 264-71.

135. Gross AR, G.C., Hoving JL, Haines T, Peloso P, Aker P, Santaguida P, Myers C, Cervical Overview Group. Conservative management of mechanical neck disorders: a systemic review. J Rheumatol, 2007. **34**(3): p. 1083-1102.

136. Woodward MN, CJ., Gargan MF, Bannister GC, Chiropractic treatment of chronic whiplash injuries. Injury, 1996. **27**: p. 643-645.

137. Fernandez-de-las-Penas C, F.-CJ., Fernandez AP, Lomas-Vega R, Miangolarra-Page JC, *Dorsal manipulation in whiplash injury treatment: a randomized controlled trial.* J Whip Rel Dis, 2004. 3: p. 55-72.

138. Paskowski I, e.a., A hospital-based standardized spine care pathway: report of multidisciplinary, evidence-based process. J Manipulative Physiol Ther., 2011. 34(2): p. 98-106.

Printed in the USA
CPSIA information can be obtained
at www.ICGtesting.com
LVHW010016130524
779591LV00001B/63